Anita Bean

Food FOR FITNESS

A & C Black • London

Food
FOR
FITNESS

Second edition

Nutrition guide • Eating plans
Over 200 recipes • Eating out guide

Anita Bean

A & C Black • London

First published 1998 by
A & C Black Publishers Ltd
37 Soho Square, London W1D 3QZ

2nd edition 2002
Reprinted 1999, 2001
Copyright © 1998, 2002 Anita Bean

ISBN 0 7136 6386 3

A CIP catalogue record for this book is available from the British
Library.

Typeset in 10.5 on 12.5pt Stempel Garamond by
Fakenham Photosetting Limited.

Note: Whilst every effort has been made to ensure that the content of
this book is as technically accurate and as sound as possible, neither
the author nor the publishers can accept responsibility for any injury
or loss sustained as a result of the use of this material.

Illustrations by Elaine Davis
Text and cover design by Jocelyn Lucas
Cover image © gettyimages

A & C Black uses paper produced with elemental chlorine-free pulp,
harvested from managed sustainable forests.

Printed and bound in Great Britain by Biddles Ltd, Guildford and
King's Lynn

Anita Bean is also the author of *The Complete Guide to Sports Nutrition:*

'*The Complete Guide to Sports Nutrition* presents an uncomplicated approach that is appropriate for all sports-active people, from the recreational exerciser to the top-level competitor. It is ideal for those who want to enhance performance and boost energy levels.'

Health and Fitness magazine

'At last, a book written by a British author which gives practical nutrition advice to all exercisers! The information in this book is relevant to EVERYONE who works out on a regular basis. It goes beyond the average 'healthy eating' recommendations that form the basis for most nutrition texts, covering the science behind the practice in a readable and interesting way.'

The Exercise Association

'*The Complete Guide to Sports Nutrition* is packed with practical advice for all levels of sport, from jogger to élite athlete. Anita Bean gives her information in a flowing style which is as easy to absorb as a hypotonic drink. I recommend this book for everyone involved in sporting performances, not only for its commonsense approach but also for its sudden insights and scattered gems of information.'

Scottish Journal of Physical Education

'This text represents good value for money. Not only does it answer numerous questions about diet, health and performance, it also provides extremely tempting recipes! This book is full of advice and sensible suggestions ... is easy to read and well presented.'

Physical Education Review

Acknowledgements

I would like to thank my husband for his invaluable support during the writing of this book, my two young daughters for their inspiration and the many sports people with whom I have worked over the years for giving me the encouragement to put pen to paper.

CONTENTS

INTRODUCTION

Food for Fitness is the practical complement to my book *The Complete Guide to Sports Nutrition* (A & C Black, 3rd edition, 2000). It is a nutrition manual, a menu planner and a recipe book all rolled into one volume. The book shows you how to work out your calorie and nutritional requirements and develop an eating plan, to enable you to get the most out of your particular training programme or sport. It is packed with hundreds of top nutrition tips, eating strategies, snack ideas and quick tasty recipes and is an essential resource for every regular exerciser!

Fitting healthy meals around a demanding training schedule is often difficult so *Food for Fitness* provides time-saving tips, easy solutions for eating on the run, ideas for quick healthy snacks, as well as an invaluable guide to the best (and worst!) fast food choices.

If you are confused about what and how much to drink when training, this book gives you the low-down on popular sports drinks, provides clear advice on preventing dehydration before, during and after exercise and gives easy recipes for home-made sports drinks.

Every sport and activity places unique nutritional demands on the athlete. I have included step-by-step eating plans for those wishing to lose body fat or gain weight, as well as detailed plans for specific athletic activities such as long distance running, swimming, cycling and sprinting.

There's nutrition advice for vegetarian athletes and those who avoid red meat. The simple diet planner will help you put together a balanced diet without meat and there's a checklist of the best foods for meat-free eating.

Food for Fitness gives you over 200 recipes to help you put the principles of sports nutrition into practice. They are all quick and easy to prepare, and make use of simple, everyday ingredients. They conform to the latest sports nutritional guidelines, being low in fat (especially saturated fats), and high in complex carbohydrates, vitamins and minerals. Most importantly, they taste delicious and have become firm favourites among my own family and athletic friends. With sections on pasta dishes, rice- and potato-based meals, one-minute meals, breakfasts, home-made breads, healthy cakes, puddings, muffins and snack bars, there's plenty to inspire even the busiest athlete or the most reluctant cook.

Anita

PART I: NUTRITION GUIDE

1 TRAINING DIET CHECKLIST

A good training diet is an essential part of every fitness programme, and will help you achieve your training and competitive goals. The right type and quantity of food will help you maintain peak health and perform at your best.

How to put together your training diet

One of the quickest and easiest ways to put together your training diet plan is to use the 'Balance of Good Health' plate model. This is based on the recommendations of the Government's *Health of the Nation* white paper, published in 1992. It is designed to meet the nutritional needs of active people. Simply balance your food choices to match the plate model shown on page 2. This features the five food groups with the number of recommended daily portions from each one. These portion goals will help you adjust your current food intake and develop a low fat, nutrient-dense eating plan that will meet your nutritional needs.

Each food group provides some, but not all, of the nutrients and energy you need. For example, milk and dairy products are rich in calcium; vitamin C is available from fruit and vegetables; and the bread, cereal and starchy vegetable group provides complex carbohydrates and fibre.

HERE'S HOW TO USE THE PLATE MODEL:

- Include foods from each group on the plate every day.
- Make sure you include a variety of foods within each group.
- Aim to have the recommended number of portions each day.
- Check the portion sizes given below.

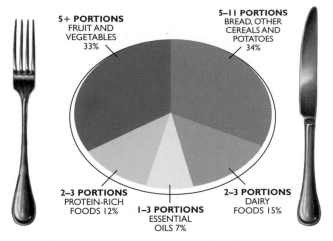

5+ PORTIONS
FRUIT AND
VEGETABLES
33%

5–11 PORTIONS
BREAD, OTHER
CEREALS AND
POTATOES
34%

2–3 PORTIONS
PROTEIN-RICH
FOODS 12%

1–3 PORTIONS
ESSENTIAL
OILS 7%

2–3 PORTIONS
DAIRY
FOODS 15%

The 'Balance of Good Health' plate model

Fruit and vegetables

Goal: minimum 5 portions

Fruit and vegetables are rich in many vitamins and minerals and are also great sources of fibre and other beneficial plant substances called phytochemicals (including the antioxidant nutrients).

How to achieve your goal:

- Include one portion of fresh fruit with your breakfast, e.g. sliced banana on breakfast cereal.
- Eat at least two portions of fresh fruit as snacks throughout the day.
- Add a side salad or crudités to your lunch or dinner.
- Include two portions of vegetables in your main meals either on their own or in soups, curries and sauces.
- Include extra salad vegetables in sandwiches.
- Follow your main meals with fresh fruit or a fruit-based dessert such as apple crumble, banana custard, baked apples, or fruit mixed with yoghurt, ice cream or rice pudding.

SIZE OF 1 PORTION	
Fresh fruit	1 apple/pear/peach/orange/banana 100 g (4 oz) berries (e.g. strawberries, raspberries) 100 g (4 oz) pineapple/grapes 4 apricots/plums 2 kiwi fruit ½ mango
Tinned fruit	½ tin (200 g) of pineapple/peaches/apricots (drained)
Fruit juice	1 glass (100 ml/3½ fl oz) juice
Vegetables	In general, 100 g (4 oz) vegetables 2 carrots/courgettes 2 florets broccoli 10 Brussels sprouts 3 tbsp peas 2–3 tbsp spinach/cabbage/runner beans
Salad	1 large tomato 7 cm (3 in) piece cucumber 1 bunch watercress 3 sticks celery 1 cos lettuce/½ iceberg lettuce

TOP TIPS

Each day aim to have:
- at least one orange/yellow fruit or vegetable (e.g. mango, apricots, carrot, tomato) for antioxidants and beta-carotene.
- at least one red fruit or vegetable (e.g. tomatoes, watermelon) for cancer-beating lycopene.
- at least one berry fruit or citrus fruit (e.g. strawberries, raspberries, oranges) for immunity-boosting bioflavanoids and vitamin C.
- at least one dark green vegetable a day (e.g. broccoli, cabbage, watercress, spinach) for iron and folic acid.

EAT MORE VEGETABLES!
Health experts recommend eating at least three portions of vegetables a day. Here are some easy ways of adding extra vegetables to your diet:

- add a handful of frozen peas or mixed vegetables to the saucepan while cooking pasta
- add extra mushrooms, peppers, aubergines, courgettes or okra to ready-made curry sauces
- keep a container of vegetable crudités (carrots, cucumber, courgette, cauliflower) in the fridge for snacking on or for starters
- add a cupful of chopped broccoli, courgettes or frozen spinach to pasta sauces
- hide puréed vegetables in soups, lasagnes, stews and pies
- make fast foods healthier by adding extra vegetables, e.g. pizza with mushrooms, peppers, tomatoes; hamburgers with tomatoes and cucumber; kebabs with extra salad; burritos with lettuce and fresh salsa.

LIVEN UP YOUR VEGETABLES
A knob of butter on your vegetables can add an extra 12 g of fat and 100 kcal. Liven up your veggies with the following fresh herbs and spices instead:

- coriander with carrots
- basil with tomatoes
- mint with peas
- thyme with peppers
- oregano with aubergine
- rosemary with leeks
- nutmeg with spinach
- dill with cabbage

Cereals and starchy vegetables

Goal: 5–11 portions (7–11 portions for active people)
This group includes bread, pasta, rice, noodles, breakfast cereals, oats, crackers, as well as starchy vegetables such as potatoes, sweet potatoes and parsnips. Foods in this group provide complex carbohydrates, B vitamins and fibre. Check your portion sizes to make sure you are eating the right amount.

How to achieve your goal:

- Start your day with at least 2–3 portions from this group, e.g. one large bowl of wholegrain cereal or porridge; 2–3 thick slices of wholemeal toast; a couple of English muffins.
- Be more adventurous with the type of bread you choose – try rye, Spanish, focaccia, ciabatta, seeded, pitta, muffins, bagels, sunflower, herb bread.
- Aim to have at least 2–3 portions of foods from this group with each meal – base meals around pasta, noodles, potatoes, rice, cous cous, bulgar wheat or bread.
- Use cooked grains, e.g. rice or bulgar, to fill vegetables such as aubergines, courgettes and peppers.

GET YOUR DAY OFF TO A HEALTHY START
Instead of grabbing a croissant and a cup of hot chocolate (331 kcal/17.1 g fat), have an English muffin with fruit spread, a banana and a glass (140 ml) of orange juice instead (330 kcal/ 1.8 g fat).

	SIZE OF 1 PORTION
Bread	1 slice bread 1 small roll/½ bap/½ bagel ½ large pitta/chappati
Cereals/grains	2 heaped tbsp cooked pasta/rice/noodles 25 g (1 oz) uncooked weight pasta/rice/noodles
Starchy vegetables	1 medium (175 g/6 oz) baked or boiled potato 3 new potatoes 2 tbsp cooked sweet potato/yam/plantain 2 tbsp sweetcorn 1 large parsnip
Breakfast cereals	1 small bowl (25 g/1 oz) breakfast cereal 2 Weetabix 1 'variety pack' box cereal
Crackers	3 crackers/crispbreads/rice cakes

TOP TIPS

- Make sure that most of your portions are wholegrain varieties, e.g. wholemeal bread/pasta, wholegrain cereal.
- Instead of butter, top jacket potatoes with fromage frais, yoghurt, cottage cheese or hummus.
- Eat baked, boiled or roast potatoes with their skin left on. There is no need to peel potatoes used in soups, stews and casseroles.

Milk and dairy products

Goal: 2–3 portions

The foods in this group – milk, cheese, yoghurt and fromage frais – are rich sources of calcium. They also provide protein, vitamin B_{12}, riboflavin and (apart from fat-free varieties) vitamins A and D. Many athletes misguidedly cut down on milk and dairy products because of their fat content, but this means missing out on other nutrients such as calcium and vitamin B_{12}. Switch to low fat varieties; they provide all the protein, minerals and water-soluble vitamins of full fat varieties, but with less fat and fat-soluble vitamins A and D.

How to achieve your goal:

- Have 200 ml (⅓ pint) milk per day (semi-skimmed or skimmed milk instead of full fat) on breakfast cereals, in drinks or puddings.
- If you don't like milk on its own, use it in shakes, custard, sauces or rice pudding.
- Aim to have one portion of cheese (preferably low fat) per day.
- Have a pot of low fat yoghurt or fromage frais for dessert.
- Use yoghurt as a base for salad dressings – add herbs, spices or lemon juice.

	SIZE OF 1 PORTION
Milk	200 ml (⅓ pint) full fat/semi-skimmed/ skimmed milk
Cheese	1 matchbox-sized piece (40 g/1 ½ oz) hard cheese (e.g. Cheddar)/soft ripened cheese (e.g. brie) 1 small pot (100 g/4 oz) cottage cheese or low fat soft cheese
Yoghurt/fromage frais	1 small pot (150 g/5 oz) yoghurt or fromage frais

TOP TIPS

- Use semi-skimmed or skimmed milk instead of full-fat.
- Limit hard (full fat) cheese to 1–2 portions per day.
- Choose low fat varieties of yoghurt/fromage frais.
- In recipes, use a strong flavoured or mature cheese so you can cut down on the amount needed.

Protein-rich foods

Goal: 2–3 portions

This group includes lean meat, chicken, turkey, fish, eggs, beans, lentils, nuts, soya and quorn. These foods supply protein, vitamins and minerals. Vegetarians can get plenty of protein from plant sources, but you may substitute extra dairy foods for one of the portions in this group.

How to achieve your goal:

- Aim to have at least half of your portions from non-meat sources.
- Use smaller amounts of meat in stews, bolognese sauce, pasta sauces, risotto, shepherds pie – substitute pulses and vegetables for some of the meat.
- Eat at least one portion of oily fish per week, e.g. mackerel, trout or sardines. The oils are rich in omega-3 fatty acids, important for preventing strokes and heart attacks, and their beneficial circulatory properties help boost exercise performance.
- Include at least three portions of pulses per week – make pulses the base for stews, curries, salads and casseroles.

- Limit processed meat (e.g. burgers, sausages) to once a week or less.

	SIZE OF 1 PORTION
Meat	2 thin slices (50–75 g/2–3 oz) red meat 1 small chop (50–75 g/2–3 oz) 3 thin slices ham
Poultry	75 g (3 oz) chicken/turkey (weighed without bone) 1 small breast
Fish	1 medium fillet (150 g/5 oz) white fish 1 small fillet (75 g/3 oz) oily fish 1 small tin (100 g/4 oz) tuna 75–100 g (3–4 oz) prawns
Eggs	2
Pulses	½ large (420 g) tin baked beans/ red kidney beans/chick peas/other beans 3 heaped tbsp cooked beans/lentils/peas
Nuts	Small handful (50 g/2 oz) nuts or seeds
Soya/tofu/quorn	100 g (4 oz) tofu/quorn 3 tbsp soya or quorn mince 1 tofu/quorn burger

TOP TIPS

- Choose lower fat foods from this group wherever possible – very lean meat, fish, poultry (without skin), pulses, eggs (up to 6 per week), quorn and soya.
- If you eat meat, make sure it is lean and well trimmed.
- If you eat poultry, remove the skin before or after cooking.
- In restaurants, order grilled fish not fried, and reduce fat by 15 g (145 kcal).
- Cook meat, fish and poultry without added fat – dry frying, grilling, baking or poaching.

Essential fats and oils

Goal: 1–3 portions

This group includes foods rich in essential oils: nuts (walnuts, cashews, almonds, pecans, brazils, pine nuts), seeds (sesame, pumpkin, sunflower), cold-pressed seed and nut oils (flax seed, pumpkin seed, walnut, sesame and sunflower), and oily fish (sardines, mackerel, pilchards, trout).

How to achieve your goal:

- A small handful of nuts or seeds eaten as a snack.
- A tablespoon of cashews or peanuts added to a stir-fry.
- A tablespoon of oil in a dressing or sauce.
- Stir a tablespoon of essential oil (e.g. flaxseed or a blended essential oil) into soup or a pasta sauce just before serving.

SIZE OF 1 PORTION	
Nuts and seeds	1 heaped tablespoon
Nut and seed oils	1 tablespoon
*Oily fish	85 g (3 oz) fish

*Oily fish is the richest source of omega-3 oils so 1–2 portions a week would more than cover your needs.

TOP TIPS

- Choose plain, unsalted nuts and avoid those with coatings or flavourings.
- Lightly toast nuts and seeds under a grill or in a hot oven for a few minutes to bring out their flavour.
- Add nuts and seeds to salads, muesli, stir-fries, crumble toppings and yoghurt.
- The nutritional value of nuts, seeds and oils is easily destroyed by heating and by exposure to light and air. So, store in dark bottles in a cool dark place.

Alcohol

The Department of Health suggests a maximum of three units per day and 14 units per week for women; and a maximum of four units per day and 21 units per week for men.

SIZE OF I UNIT
250 ml (½ pint) ordinary strength beer/lager I small glass (125 ml/4 fl oz) wine I single measure sherry/vermouth I single measure spirits

TOP TIPS

- Have at least two alcohol-free days per week.
- Pace your drinking – alternate low calorie soft drinks with alcoholic drinks, or mix dry white wine and sparkling water or soda water to make your drink last longer.
- Keep a tally on your alcohol intake when you go out – set yourself a safe limit.
- Don't nibble salty snacks with your alcoholic drink – they will make you more thirsty.
- Extend your alcoholic drink (e.g. wine, spirits) with water, low calorie mixers or soda water, or alternate alcoholic and non-alcoholic drinks.
- If you think you have drunk too much, drink plenty of water/sports drink before retiring to bed – at least one pint per 2–3 units.
- Do not feel obliged to drink excessively even if your friends press you. Tell them you are training the next day or that you are driving.
- Do not drink on an empty stomach as this speeds alcohol absorption. Try to eat something first or reserve drinking for meal times. Food slows down the absorption of alcohol.
- To minimise a hangover, choose pale-coloured drinks (e.g. white wine) rather than dark drinks; avoid carbonated alcoholic drinks (e.g. gin & tonic, champagne) as the alcohol is absorbed faster.

> **DID YOU KNOW**
> Cutting down – but not giving up – on your alcohol intake can help you lose unwanted body fat. One glass of wine is equivalent to 95 kcal so if you reduce your intake by seven glasses of wine per week, you'll save 2660 kcal a month, that's nearly ½ kg (1 lb) of body fat!

Fatty and sugary foods

Goal: up to 1 portion
This group includes biscuits, cakes, sweets, soft drinks, chocolate, puddings and crisps. These supply lots of calories with very few (if any) essential nutrients ('empty calories').

How to achieve your goal

- Regard fatty and sugary foods as treats rather than everyday foods.
- Limit high fat puddings and cakes to three times per week or less.
- Limit salty/sugary snacks to three times per week or less.

SIZE OF 1 PORTION

1 packet crisps	1 slice cake
3 biscuits	1 chocolate/confectionery bar

TOP TIPS

Substitute the following low fat snacks for high fat snacks:
- sandwiches/rolls/pitta/bagels (filled with cottage cheese/peanut butter/banana/salad/honey/marmite/tuna/chicken/turkey/ham)
- low fat yoghurt and fromage frais
- fresh fruit (e.g. apples, bananas, nectarines, grapes)
- English muffins/scones/crumpets/potato cakes
- dried fruit
- dried fruit bars/'energy' bars/cereal bars/protein bars
- nuts and dried fruit mixtures
- rice cakes/crackers/bread sticks.

DID YOU KNOW?

One packet of crisps contains 11 g fat (about 2 tsp) and 160 kcal – that's 62% of calories from fat! Switching to reduced fat crisps is a step in the right direction but they are still high in salt. Better substitutes include:

- 1 cup (15 g) of plain popcorn (55 kcal/0.3 g fat)
- 5 bread sticks (100 kcal/0.5 g fat)
- 3 rice cakes (75 kcal/0.3 g fat).

DID YOU KNOW?

Carob bars are *not* a low fat alternative to chocolate. Although they contain no caffeine, most brands contain more fat and the same amount of sugar as ordinary plain chocolate and cost considerably more.

References

1 *The National Food Guide*, Health Education Authority in partnership with the Dept of Health and MAFF, July 1994
2 *Nutritional Aspects of Cardiovascular Disease*, COMA, HMSO, November 1994

2 THE CARBOHYDRATE CONNECTION

Carbohydrates are the number one fuel for energy for virtually every activity and sport, and should supply around 60% of your calorie intake. They are also needed to fuel the brain and other vital functions in the body. A high carbohydrate diet gives you the following benefits.

INCREASED STAMINA
High levels of stored carbohydrate (glycogen) in the muscles allows you to exercise longer before feeling exhausted. Low glycogen stores result in early fatigue. While fat and protein can also provide fuel during aerobic (cardiovascular) activities, it is carbohydrate only that is burned during the earlier stage of exercise and also during anaerobic (very high-intensity, explosive) activities. Carbohydrate is therefore the best fuel for increasing stamina.

INCREASED PERFORMANCE
High glycogen levels help you to maintain a higher training intensity for longer and so improve your sports performance. This is important for all types of activities. Studies prove that athletes on high carbohydrate diets (i.e. above 60% of calorie intake) achieve significantly better results compared with those on low carbohydrate diets.

GOOD FOR HEALTH
Many foods rich in carbohydrates, such as cereals, bread, rice and potatoes also contain B vitamins for a healthy nervous system and efficient energy production, fibre for healthy digestion, and iron for healthy blood. Fruit, also high in carbohydrates, is an excellent source of vitamin C for immunity and other antioxidants that fight cancer and heart disease.

How much carbohydrate?

To work out how much carbohydrate you need each day, multiply your weight (in kg) by the corresponding figure shown in the table.

ACTIVITY LEVEL*	CARBOHYDRATE IN g/kg BODY WEIGHT PER DAY
2–5 hours/week	4–5
5–7 hours/week	5–6
1–2 hours/day	6–7
2–4 hours/day	7–8
more than 4 hours/day	8–10

*Activity levels take account of both duration and intensity of activity. The time refers to the hours of continuous activity (i.e. not including rest periods).

For example, if you weigh 60 kg and you exercise for 1–2 hours per day:

Carbohydrate needs = (60 × 6) to (60 × 7) = 360 to 420 g per day

To give you an idea of how much food you should eat, you could get 400 g carbohydrate from:

- 17 bananas, or
- 27 slices of toast, or
- 14 baked potatoes, or
- 40 biscuits, or
- 2 rolls, 2 slices of toast, 2 baked potatoes, 2 apples, 1 small tin (200 g/7 oz) of baked beans, 1 generous portion (75 g/ 3 oz) of pasta, 2 bananas, 2 cartons fruit yoghurt, ½ pint semi-skimmed milk and 1 fruit scone.

Use the carbohydrate counter opposite to work out how much food you should eat.

THE CARBOHYDRATE COUNTER

FOOD	PORTION	CARBOHYDRATE (TOTAL) (g)
Bread and cereals		
Rice (white)	100 g uncooked	87
Pasta	100 g uncooked	76
Pitta bread	1 pitta (75 g)	43
Bran Flakes	large bowl (60 g)	42
Muesli	medium bowl (50 g)	33
Roll	1 roll (48 g)	23
Porridge oats	3 tbsp (30 g)	20
Weetabix	1 Weetabix (20 g)	15
Bread	1 slice (36 g)	15
Crispbread	1 crispbread (10 g)	7.1
Cracker	1 cracker (7 g)	5.8
Potatoes/ vegetables		
Baked beans	half a tin (200 g)	30
Baked potato	medium (160 g)	29
Sweetcorn	3 tbsp (85 g)	23
Crisps	1 bag (30 g)	16
Cakes/ desserts/ biscuits		
Fruit cake	1 slice (70 g)	42
Flapjack	1 flapjack (70 g)	42
Sponge cake	1 slice (60 g)	39
Currant bun	1 bun (60 g)	32
Ice cream	2 scoops (85 g)	17
Digestive biscuit	1 biscuit (15 g)	10
Confectionery/ sugars		
Mars Bar	standard bar (65 g)	43
Cola	1 can (340 g)	37
Milk chocolate	small bar (54 g)	31
Jam/marmalade	1 tbsp (15 g)	10
Sugar	1 tsp (6 g)	6

FOOD	PORTION	CARBOHYDRATE (TOTAL) (g)
Dairy products		
Milk	1 pint (585 g)	29
Fruit yoghurt	1 carton (150 g)	27
Cheddar cheese	matchbox-size (40 g)	0
Fruit		
Banana	1 large banana (100 g)	23
Raisins	1 handful (30 g)	21
Orange juice	1 glass (160 g)	14
Apple/pear/orange	1 piece of fruit (100 g)	12

Eating after exercise

It takes a minimum of 20 hours to fully replenish carbohydrate stores. During the first two hours after exercise, glycogen is restored at a faster rate than normal (almost one and a half times faster). So consuming carbohydrate during this time will speed up overall recovery. This is particularly important if you exercise daily or even twice daily.

Aim to consume 1 g carbohydrate per kg body weight within two hours of training. For example, if you weigh 60 kg you need to consume approximately 60 g of carbohydrate during this period.

The best types of carbohydrates are those which are absorbed rapidly into the body; both solid and liquid forms are equally effective. Many athletes prefer taking a drink such as diluted juice, squash or a sports drink. This has the advantage of also providing fluid.

BEST SNACKS (APPROX. 60 g CARBOHYRDRATE)

- 1 energy bar
- 2 large bananas
- 3 handfuls raisins
- 4 slices bread or toast (plain)
- 2 slices bread or toast with 2 tbsp jam
- 2 fruit bars/cereal bars
- 8 rice cakes or crispbreads
- 1 litre isotonic sports drink (6% carbohydrate)
- 200 ml squash diluted with 800 ml water

Eating before exercise

Don't exercise on a full stomach nor when your stomach is completely empty. As a general rule of thumb allow:

- 3–4 hours for a large meal to digest
- 2–3 hours for a small–medium meal to digest
- approximately one hour for a snack to digest

The benefits of a pre-exercise meal or snack include:

- preventing hunger pangs and settling the stomach
- fuelling the muscles and improving performance
- preventing low blood sugar levels (hypoglycaemia)

BEST PRE-EXERCISE MEALS

The pre-exercise meal should have a moderate–low glycaemic index (see page 20) and be relatively low in fat.

- Porridge with fruit
- Breakfast cereal with milk
- Pasta with chicken and vegetables
- Rice with beans and salad
- Low fat cheese or tuna sandwich
- Baked potato with beans, tuna or cheese

BEST PRE-EXERCISE SNACKS (SUPPLYING 25 g CARBOHYDRATE)

- 2 portions of fresh fruit
- 400 ml isotonic sports drink (6% carbohydrate)
- 1 large handful raisins
- 1 slice bread with jam or honey
- 1 cereal or fruit bar
- Low-fat muffin (see recipes pages 225–228)

Eating during exercise

If you are exercising hard for more than 90 minutes, you can delay fatigue by consuming additional carbohydrate (in solid or liquid form) during exercise. Most studies show that 30–60 g carbohydrate per hour helps maintain blood sugar levels, delay glycogen depletion and improve endurance. Start consuming carbohydrate after about 30 minutes and continue at regular intervals until the end of your training session. If you have solid forms of carbohydrate such as energy bars or gels, drink plain water rather than a sports drink.

BEST SNACKS AND DRINKS DURING EXERCISE* (SUPPLYING 30 g PER HOUR)

- 500 ml isotonic sports drink (6% carbohydrate)
- 500 ml diluted fruit juice (1:1)
- 1 energy bar (plus 500 ml water)
- Energy gel (plus 500 ml water)
- 1½ handfuls dried fruit (plus 500 ml water)

At higher exercise intensities, double the quantities.

Eating between workouts

Eat at regular intervals throughout the day to ensure efficient refuelling between hard training sessions. Eating 'little and often' also keeps up your energy levels, maintains a steady blood sugar concentration and minimises body fat storage. Leaving long gaps between meals results in plummeting energy levels, incomplete glycogen refuelling and a lower nutrient intake. Aim to eat 3–4 moderate-sized meals and top up your energy levels throughout the day with 2–3 nutritious snacks.

Fast and slow carbs – the Glycaemic index (GI)

Some carbohydrates are quickly absorbed, producing a rapid rise in blood sugar. These foods give a quick energy boost. Others are absorbed more slowly, producing a smaller but more prolonged rise in blood glucose.

The ability of a food to raise blood sugar levels is measured by its **glycaemic index (GI).**

High glycaemic index foods (e.g. bananas, sugar, potatoes, rice) produce a rapid rise in blood sugar. These foods are quickly digested and absorbed giving a quick energy boost, and are readily converted into energy or glycogen. Foods with a high GI are advantageous to performance during and immediately after exercise.

Low glycaemic index foods (e.g. pulses, oats, most fruit) produce a slower blood sugar rise so the carbohydrate becomes available more slowly. These foods are best eaten 2–4 hours before exercise because they produce more sustained energy, and also in-between exercise sessions to promote efficient glycogen refuelling.

Combining foods with high and low GIs (e.g. cheese and bread) results in an intermediate GI. In general, protein and fat reduce the speed of carbohydrate absorption and therefore reduce the GI. For example, plain bread produces a rapid blood sugar rise, desirable immediately before or after exercise; adding a layer of butter or a slice of cheese slows the blood sugar rise, desirable during the refuelling period.

THE GLYCAEMIC INDEX AND CARBOHYDRATE CONTENT OF FOODS

FOOD	PORTION SIZE	GI	CARBOHYDRATE (g)
Breakfast cereals			
Muesli	small bowl (50 g)	56	34
Weetabix	2 (40 g)	69	30
Shredded wheat	2 (45 g)	67	31
Rice crispies	small bowl (30 g)	82	27
Cornflakes	small bowl (30 g)	84	26
Cheerios	small bowl (30 g)	74	23
Porridge (made with water)	small bowl (160 g)	42	14
Grains/pasta			
Rice — brown	6 tbsp (180 g)	76	58
Rice — white	6 tbsp (180 g)	87	56
Spaghetti	4 tbsp (220 g cooked)	41	49
Rice — basmati	4 tbsp (60 g)	58	48
Pasta — macaroni	4 tbsp (230 g cooked)	45	43
Noodles — instant	4 tbsp (230 g cooked)	46	30
Bread			
Pizza	1 large slice (115 g)	60	38
White bread	1 large slice (36 g)	70	18
Wholemeal bread	1 large slice (38 g)	69	16
Crackers/Crispbreads			
Rice cakes	1 (8 g)	85	6
Biscuits and cakes			
Sponge cake	1 slice (60 g)	46	39
Muffin	1 (68 g)	44	34
Digestive	1 (15 g)	59	10
Shortbread	1 (13 g)	64	8
Oatmeal	1 (13 g)	55	8
Rich tea	1 (10 g)	55	8

FOOD	PORTION SIZE	GI	CARBOHYDRATE (g)
Vegetables			
Chips	average portion (165 g)	75	59
Potato – boiled, old	2 medium (175 g)	56	30
Potato — mashed	4 tbsp (180 g)	70	28
Sweet potato	1 medium (130 g)	54	27
Potato — boiled, new	7 small (175 g)	62	27
Potato — jacket	1 average (180 g)	85	22
Sweetcorn	2 tbsp (85 g)	55	17
Parsnip	2 tbsp (65 g)	97	8
Peas	2 tbsp (70 g)	48	7
Carrots	2 tbsp (60 g)	49	3
Pulses			
Baked beans	1 small tin (205 g)	48	31
Lentils (red)	4 tbsp (160 g)	26	28
Chickpeas	4 tbsp (140 g)	33	24
Red kidney beans	4 tbsp (120 g)	27	20
Fruit			
Banana	1 (100 g)	55	23
Raisins	1 tbsp (30 g)	64	21
Pear	1 (160 g)	38	16
Apricot (dried)	5 (40 g)	31	15
Grapes	small bunch (100 g)	46	15
Apple	1 (100 g)	38	12
Orange	1 (208 g)	44	12
Mango	½ (75 g)	55	11
Cherries	small handful (100 g)	22	10
Pineapple	1 slice (80 g)	66	8
Peach	1 (121 g)	42	8
Kiwi fruit	1 (68 g)	52	6
Plum	1 (55 g)	39	5
Apricot	1 (40 g)	57	3
Drinks			
Fanta	375 ml can	68	51
Lucozade	250 ml bottle	95	40
Isostar	250 ml can	70	18
Squash (diluted)	250 ml glass		
	(from 50 ml concentrate)	66	14
Snacks			
Tortillas/corn chips	1 bag (50 g)	72	30
Crisps	1 packet (30 g)	54	16
Peanuts	small handful (50 g)	14	4
Dairy products			
Yoghurt, fruit (low-fat)	1 pot (150 g)	33	27
Milk — skimmed	½ pint (300 ml)	32	15
Milk — whole	½ pint (300 ml)	27	14
Ice cream	1 scoop (60 g)	61	14
Confectionery			
Mars bar	1 standard (65 g)	68	43
Milk chocolate	1 bar (54 g)	49	31
Muesli bar	1 (33 g)	61	20
Drinks			
Apple juice	1 glass (160 ml)	40	16
Orange juice	1 glass (160 ml)	46	14
Sugars			
Honey	1 heaped tsp (17 g)	58	13
Glucose	1 tsp (5 g)	100	5
Sucrose	1 tsp (5 g)	65	5

Note: 60–100 = high GI, 40–60 = moderate GI, < 40 = low GI.

3 FAT COUNTER

A small amount of fat is essential for health, but the average person's intake is greatly in excess of this. Regular exercisers should consume between 15 and 30% of their calories as fat. As fat has more than twice as many calories as carbohydrate or protein (9 kcal/g compared with 4 kcal/g) it is easy to consume a lot of calories in only a small amount of food.

WHY FAT MAKES YOU FAT

The fat you eat is readily converted into body fat. It takes far fewer calories to metabolise fat than carbohydrate or protein, so you are more likely to accumulate body fat on a high fat diet than a high carbohydrate diet containing the same number of calories.

Fat does not satisfy the appetite as well as carbohydrate or protein so it is easy to overeat fatty foods without feeling full. Numerous studies have shown that diets with a high percentage of fat result in increased fat accumulation.

Too much fat (especially saturated fat) increases the risk of obesity, heart disease and certain types of cancer. Also, a high fat diet is likely to be too low in carbohydrate and can therefore leave your muscles underfuelled.

Low fat, not no fat!

An entirely fat-free diet is not desirable either and a minimum of 15% calories from fat is recommended. This allows you to:

- get adequate essential fatty – the omega-3 and omega-6 fatty acids – needed for prostaglandin (hormone-like substances) manufacture, tissue growth, cell membranes and healthy

skin. They are found in vegetable oils, nuts, seeds and oily
fish
- obtain the fat-soluble vitamins A, D and E
- make vitamin A from beta-carotene
- absorb and transport fat-soluble vitamins in the body
- enjoy a palatable diet and include a wide range of foods
  without the guilt! Fat adds to the flavour and texture of
  many foods.

Aim to get between 15 and 30% of your calories from fat. How much
fat does this translate into? For example, if you consume 2500 kcal a
day, 25% calories from fat equals 625 kcal. Since 1 g of fat provides
9 kcal, that gives you a daily allowance of 625 ÷ 9 = 69 g of fat. The
chart below shows how 25% of calories from fat translates into grams
of fat depending on your calorie intake.

CALORIE INTAKE	FAT (g)
1500	42
2000	56
2500	69
3000	83
3500	97
4000	111

It is best to choose fats with the greatest health benefits – foods containing more polyunsaturated and monounsaturated fatty acids than
saturated fatty acids (see pages 25–6). Keep foods high in saturated
fatty acids to a minimum.

Most people need to reduce their overall fat intake and saturated
fatty acids in particular. A low fat diet can be achieved by:

- minimising the addition of fat to your food – use less butter
  and spreads, dressings and cooking oil
- choosing reduced fat dairy products, such as low fat milk
  and cheeses
- avoiding high fat snack foods such as crisps, chocolate and
  cakes
- choosing lean cuts of meat and substituting skinless poultry,
  white fish or pulses for some of the meat in your diet.

Fats in your food

WORST CHOICES
Saturated fatty acids
These are solid fats, mostly of animal origin, that encourage the body to produce more LDL (bad) cholesterol. Associated with a higher cancer risk.
Sources: meat, lard, butter, dairy products (except skimmed milk), products containing palm and coconut oil (e.g. hard margarine, biscuits and processed snacks).

Trans fatty acids
These are polyunsaturates artificially hardened by adding extra hydrogen. They are as bad or more harmful than saturates; they increase LDL cholesterol and heart disease risk, and lower HDL (good) cholesterol.
Sources: hard margarine, products containing hydrogenated vegetable fats, e.g. biscuits, cakes.

GOOD CHOICES
Polyunsaturated fatty acids
Polyunsaturates are liquid oils mainly from plant sources or oily fish. They are better than saturates as they lower total and LDL cholesterol levels and so reduce heart disease risk, however they also reduce HDL cholesterols.
Sources: vegetable, seed and nut oils, margarine and other products made from these oils, oily fish.

Essential fatty acids
These are a sub-group of polyunsaturates which are essential for health but cannot be made by the body. They are used for making cell membranes and hormone-like substances called prostaglandins which regulate many body processes. The two main EFAs are linoleic acid (an omega-6 fatty acid) and linolenic acid (an omega-3 fatty acid).

Omega-6 fatty acids
These polyunsaturated fatty acids include linoleic acid and its derivatives. They reduce LDL (bad) cholesterol, but at very high intakes may also reduce HDL (good) cholesterol. High intakes may also encourage increased free radical damage and, therefore, increase the risk of cancer. A moderate intake is recommended.
Sources: vegetable oils, polyunsaturated margarine, products made from these oils.

BEST CHOICES
Monounsaturated fatty acids
These are liquid at room temperature but solidify when chilled. Replacing saturates with monounsaturates reduces the risk of heart disease. They can reduce LDL (bad) cholesterol but maintain HDL (good) cholesterol, and appear to reduce free radical damage associated with certain cancers, heart disease and rheumatoid arthritis.
Sources: olive oil, rapeseed oil, nut oils, avocados, nuts and seeds.

Omega-3 fatty acids
These polyunsaturated fatty acids include linolenic acid and its derivatives. These long chain derivatives reduce the risk of thrombosis (blood clots) and, therefore, heart attacks and strokes. They also help to control inflammation and reduce the risk of inflammatory diseases such as rheumatoid arthritis.
Sources: oily fish, walnuts, linseeds, dark green leafy vegetables.

HIDDEN FATS

It's easy to cut down on visible fat such as butter, margarine, the fat on meat, the skin on poultry, cream, and the oil you cook in. However, much of the fat we eat is hidden inside foods such as biscuits, cakes, sauces, savoury snack foods and fast foods. The fat finder opposite will help you to recognise some of these sources and choose your foods more wisely.

FAT FINDER

VERY LOW FAT FOODS (<2% FAT)   FAT CONTENT (g/100 g)

Sugar	0
Jam	0
Cola	0
Egg white	0
Skimmed milk	0.1
Quark	0.1
Apples	0.1
Potatoes	0.1
White fish/tuna tinned in brine	0.2
Low calorie yoghurt	0.2
Bananas	0.3
Carrots	0.4
Baked beans	0.6
Pasta	0.7
Broccoli	0.8
Low fat yoghurt	0.8
Rice	1.3
White bread	1.9
Bran flakes	1.9

LOW FAT FOODS (2–5% FAT)

Semi-skimmed milk	2.8
Whole milk yoghurt	3
Cottage cheese	3.9
Chicken breast	5
Fillet steak (extra lean)	5

MEDIUM FAT FOODS (6–20% FAT)

Muesli	6
Ice cream	10
Eggs	11
Beef (regular cut)	12
Bacon (lean)	13
Minced beef	14
Muesli (deluxe)	14
Plain biscuits	17
Sausages (grilled)	17

HIGH FAT FOODS (21–40% FAT)	
Chocolate biscuits	24
Sponge cake	26
Shortbread	26
Pastry	28
Reduced fat mayonnaise	28
Chocolate	31
Cheddar cheese	34
Whipping cream	39
VERY HIGH FAT FOODS (41–100% FAT)	
Low fat spread	41
Peanuts	53
French dressing	72
Mayonnaise	76
Margarine	82
Butter	82
Sunflower/olive oil	100

HOW MUCH FAT?

Here's the fat content of some popular foods and snacks.

Cheese and tomato pizza	35 g
Quarter pounder with cheese	26 g
1 tbsp mayonnaise	23 g
1 slice chocolate cake	21 g
Small portion of chips	20 g
1 flapjack	19 g
1 slice of cheese (40 g)	14 g
Chocolate bar	12 g
1 croissant	10 g
1 packet of crisps	10 g
2 chocolate biscuits	9 g
1 knob of butter	8 g
1 cereal bar	8 g
2 sausages (2 × 20 g)	8 g

TWELVE WAYS TO CUT FAT IN YOUR COOKING

1 Use as little oil or butter as possible when cooking. Instead of frying, use other methods which involve very little or no added fat, such as grilling, boiling, baking, microwaving, or barbecuing on an open grill plate.

2 Use a non-stick frying pan, brush lightly with oil or use an oil spray before cooking.

3 When preparing soups and casseroles, pre-cook onions or vegetables in a little passata (smooth sieved tomatoes) or vegetable stock.

4 Reduce the amount of meat needed in casseroles, bolognese sauces and stews by adding extra beans or vegetables; cooked aubergine flesh or chestnut mushrooms provide a 'meaty' texture.

5 Cook meat, poultry or fish en papillote ('in a bag'). Simply encase in either greaseproof paper or foil along with herbs or spices and chopped vegetables so the meat/fish steam-roasts within the bag.

6 Trim all the visible fat from meat and remove the skin from poultry. Choose cuts of meat with the least marbling.

7 Substitute two egg whites for one whole egg when baking cakes and puddings.

8 Use low fat Greek yoghurt, fromage blanc or quark in place of cream for making 'creamy' sauces. Unlike ordinary yoghurt, these ingredients can all be heated without curdling.

9 Marinate meat and chicken before cooking to improve tenderness and flavour. You will then need to add less or no fat when cooking.

10 For salads, modify the usual oil/vinegar dressings by diluting with water or extra vinegar or using less oil. Substitute mayonnaise with yoghurt or fromage frais-based dressings (see pages 127–8).

11 Make 'pastry' cases from ordinary bread slices moulded into bun tins and baked for 15–20 mins at 150° C/300° F/gas mark 2 until dried through. These are perfect for filling with spreads and dips.

12 Stir frying is an excellent way to cook foods quickly in minimal quantities of oil. Allow one tablespoon per 450 g (1 lb) of vegetables.

LOW FAT SWAPS

HIGH FAT INGREDIENT	LOW FAT ALTERNATIVES
Shortcrust/puff pastry	Filo pastry; bread dough (see page 166); line pie dish/muffin tins with thin slices of bread; potato pastry (see page 187); vegetable pie crust (see page 188).
Margarine/butter in cakes	For each 100 g (4 oz) fat, substitute 175 g (6 oz) prunes puréed with 4 tbsp water or 175 g (6 oz) mixture of apricots, dates and prunes puréed with 4 tsp water or fruit juice.
Margarine/butter in white sauce	Omit fat. Blend 1 heaped tbsp cornflour with 250 ml (½ pint) milk.
Cream	Greek yoghurt (standard or low fat); low fat yoghurt; fromage blanc; half fat crème fraîche; quark; evaporated skimmed milk; lightly beaten soft tofu.
Cheddar cheese	Smaller quantity of strong flavoured cheese; for topping use half grated cheese and half breadcrumbs or oats.
Cream cheese	Ricotta cheese; quark (blended with a little sugar and vanilla essence in sweet dishes).

4 VITAMINS AND MINERALS

Vitamins are vital for energy production, growth and overall health. Minerals are also needed for energy production as well as healthy bones and teeth, muscle contraction and fluid balance.

Regular exercise increases the requirements for most vitamins and minerals, however most athletes can meet these needs from a balanced diet. There is usually a direct relationship between food intake and vitamins – the more you eat the more vitamins and minerals you will take in.

To supplement or not?

Many athletes take vitamin and mineral supplements in the belief that they will lead to better performance. The vast majority of research has found that vitamin deficiencies adversely affect performance, but excessive intakes will not improve it. Large doses of certain vitamins and minerals may be harmful and interfere with the absorption of other nutrients in the diet.

Many people take a simple multi-vitamin and mineral supplement as an 'insurance policy' to ensure they are getting enough. As intense exercise increases the requirements for many vitamins and minerals, this may be a good strategy. However, supplements should not replace a healthy diet; no vitamin or mineral will compensate for a high fat or low calorie/carbohydrate intake.

WHO NEEDS THEM?

You may benefit from taking supplements if you are:

Dieting. Restricting your calories below 1500 kcal a day will result in deficient intakes of certain nutrients.
Eating an erratic diet. Certain lifestyles, e.g. travelling, shift working, can make it difficult to eat a balanced diet.

Pregnant. Requirements of several vitamins and minerals increase during pregnancy. Folic acid supplements (0.4 mg per day) are recommended prior to pregnancy and during the first 12 weeks of pregnancy in order to reduce the risk of neural tube defects such as spina bifida.

Allergic to certain foods. People who have to omit major food groups (dairy products, wheat products) need to consume alternative sources of certain nutrients or take supplements. (Consult your doctor or dietician.)

A vegan. Those people who eat no animal products may have deficient intakes of calcium, iron, riboflavin and vitamin B_{12} and may benefit from supplements.

A heavy smoker. Smoking has an adverse effect on athletic performance and health and depletes the body's vitamin C levels, so a supplement may help compensate for this.

Antioxidant foods

An antioxidant-rich diet may help protect against heart disease and cancer, delay ageing and promote faster recovery after exercise. Antioxidants – which neutralise the effects of free radicals – include vitamins (beta-carotene, vitamin C, vitamin E), minerals (such as selenium and zinc), and plant compounds called phytochemicals. In general, you'll find them in plant foods: fruit and vegetables, seeds, nuts, oils, whole grains, beans and lentils.

TOP ANTIOXIDANT-RICH FRUIT AND VEGETABLES
Researchers at Tufts University have compiled a league table of fruits and vegetables according to their antioxidant power:

1. Prunes
2. Raisins
3. Blueberries
4. Blackberries
5. Garlic
6. Curly kale
7. Strawberries
8. Raspberries
9. Spinach
10. Brussels sprouts
11. Plums
12. Red peppers
13. Broccoli

Here are the best food sources of other antioxidants:

Vitamin C	Citrus fruit, berries, peppers
Vitamin E	Sunflower and nut oils, avocado, almonds, salmon
Selenium	Brazil nuts, meat, whole grains
Beta-carotene	Carrots, apricots, red peppers, mango
Flavanoids	Fruit, vegetables, tea, garlic, red wine
Lycopene	Tomatoes, watermelon

KEEP THE VITAMINS IN!

- Buy fresh, firm fruit and vegetables; avoid bruised, soft or wilted produce.
- Keep vegetables in a cool dark place, such as the salad compartment in the fridge.
- Don't prepare food too far in advance – vitamins are lost if cut up fruit or vegetables are left to stand.
- Keep the skin or peel on wherever possible as most vitamins are found just beneath the surface.
- Cut into large pieces rather than small; vitamins are lost from cut surfaces.
- Cook vegetables in the minimum amount of water – steaming, microwaving or stir frying retains more vitamins.
- Make sure water is fast-boiling before adding vegetables.
- Cook vegetables for as little time as possible until they are tender-crisp.
- Save the cooking water for soup, stock and sauces.

THE ESSENTIAL VITAMINS AND MINERALS GUIDE

VITAMIN	RDA*	FUNCTIONS	SOURCES
A	700 ug (men) 600 ug (women)	Vision in dim light; maintains healthy skin and linings of the digestive tract, nose and throat.	Full fat dairy products; meat; offal; oily fish; margarine.
Beta-carotene	No official RDA, 15–25 mg suggested	Antioxidant which protects against certain cancers; converts into vitamin A.	Fruit and vegetables, e.g. apricots, peppers, tomatoes, mangoes, broccoli.
B₁ (Thiamin)	1 mg (men) 0.8 mg (women) OR 0.4 mg/1000 kcal	Releases energy from carbohydrates; maintains healthy nervous system and digestive system.	Wholemeal bread and cereals; pulses; meat.

33

VITAMIN	RDA*	FUNCTIONS	SOURCES
B_2 (Riboflavin)	1.3 mg (men) 1.1 mg (women)	Releases energy from carbohydrates; maintains healthy skin, eyes and nerves.	Milk and dairy products; meat; eggs.
B_3 (Niacin)	17 mg (men) 13 mg (women) OR 6.6 mg/1000 kcal	Releases energy from carbohydrates; maintains healthy skin, nerves and digestion.	Meat and offal; nuts; milk and dairy products; eggs; wholegrain cereals.
B_6 (Pyridoxine)	1.4 mg (men) 1.2 mg (women)	Metabolism of protein, carbohydrate, fat; red blood cell manufacture; maintains healthy immune system.	Pulses; nuts; eggs; cereals; fish; bananas.
Pantothenic acid	No official RDA	Metabolism of protein, carbohydrate, fat; maintains healthy skin, hair and immune system.	Wholegrain cereals; nuts; pulses; eggs; vegetables.
Folic acid	200 ug (+ 400 ug in pregnancy)	Formation of DNA and red blood cells; reduces risk of spina bifida in developing babies.	Green leafy vegetables; yeast extract; pulses.

VITAMIN	RDA*	FUNCTIONS	SOURCES
B_{12}	1.5 ug	Formation of red blood cells; energy metabolism.	Milk and dairy products; meat; fish; fortified breakfast cereals, soya products and yeast extract.
C	40 mg	Maintains healthy connective tissue, bones, teeth, blood vessels, gums and teeth; promotes immune function; helps iron absorption.	Fruit and vegetables, e.g. raspberries, blackcurrants, kiwi, oranges, peppers, broccoli, cabbage, tomatoes.
D	No official RDA (10 ug recommended in pregnancy)	Builds strong bones; needed to absorb calcium and phosphorus.	Sunlight; oily fish; fortified margarine and breakfast cereals; eggs.
E	No official RDA in UK (10 mg in EU)	Antioxidant which works against heart disease; promotes normal cell growth and development.	Vegetable oils; oily fish; nuts; seeds; egg yolk; avocado.

MINERAL	RDA*	FUNCTIONS	SOURCES
Calcium	700 mg	Builds bone and teeth; blood clotting; nerve and muscle function.	Milk and dairy products; sardines; dark green leafy vegetables; pulses; nuts and seeds.
Iron	8.7 mg (men) 14.8 mg (women)	Formation of red blood cells; oxygen transport; prevents anaemia.	Meat and offal; wholegrain cereals; fortified breakfast cereals; pulses; green leafy vegetables.
Zinc	9.5 mg (men) 7 mg (women)	Healthy immune system; wound healing; healthy skin; cell growth.	Eggs; wholegrain cereals; meat; milk and dairy products.
Magnesium	300 mg (men) 270 ug (women)	Healthy bones; muscle and nerve function; cell formation.	Cereals; fruit; vegetables; milk.
Potassium	3.5 mg	Fluid balance; muscle and nerve function.	Fruit; vegetables; cereals.
Sodium	1.6 mg	Fluid balance; muscle and nerve function.	Salt; processed meat; ready meals; sauces; soup; cheese; bread.
Selenium	0.9 ug (men) 0.8 ug (women)	Antioxidant which helps protect against heart disease and cancer.	Cereals; vegetables; dairy products; meat; eggs.

*RDA = recommended daily amount

CHOOSING A MULTIVITAMIN/MINERAL SUPPLEMENT

- Choose a full spectrum supplement that contains at least 23 vitamins and minerals.
- Some vitamins and minerals can be toxic in excess – take no more than the RDA for minerals and no more than 10 × the RDA for vitamins A and D (the B vitamins and vitamins C and E are considered safe in higher doses).
- Do not exceed the manufacturer's recommended dose.
- Lower dose supplements designed to be taken in two or more daily doses are safer than mega doses.
- Choose food-form supplements, which contain nutrients in their natural food structure and so are better absorbed by the body.
- Always seek professional advice for a correct diagnosis about any symptoms you experience.

5 BULKING UP

Gains in strength and muscle size involve a balance of diet and training. Simply eating more food will not increase your muscle bulk unless you follow a sensible weight training programme. Similarly, spending hours in the gym will not produce the results you want unless you change your diet.

Bulking up – the formula for success

STEP 1: TRAINING

- Obtain a professionally planned weight training programme. This should include 1–3 different exercises for each body part; 3–4 sets and 6–10 repetitions of each exercise.
- Intermediate and advanced trainers should use a split training system so each body part is trained once every 5–7 days. Get plenty of rest between workouts so your muscles are fully recovered and refuelled.
- Aim to complete each workout in about 45 minutes.
- Ensure you use strict technique – perform each repetition through the full range of movement in a controlled manner. Avoid 'cheating', e.g. swinging the weight, performing incomplete movements or using too heavy a weight for your ability.

STEP 2: INCREASE YOUR CALORIE INTAKE

- Increase your calorie intake by 15–20%. If you normally consume 2500 kcal a day, add an extra 375–500 kcal.
- Divide your food intake into three meals and at least 2–3 nutritious snacks. Avoid leaving longer than four hours between eating.
- Get organised, prepare meals in advance and take snacks with you so you always have suitable food to hand.

- If you find it difficult to eat enough food, supplement your food intake with liquid meals (home-made milkshakes or carbohydrate/protein meal replacement supplements), reduce your fibre intake, and include more energy-dense snacks.

STEP 3: GET THE RIGHT BALANCE OF CARBOHYDRATE, PROTEIN AND FAT

- Eat enough carbohydrate (around 60% of your calorie intake). Your body will break down protein (muscle) if your carbohydrate intake is too low.
- Consume between 1.4 and 1.8 g protein/kg body weight per day. Include a portion of a protein-rich food with each meal.
- Don't go overboard on protein; excess is simply converted into glycogen or fat.
- Keep your fat intake low (less than 30% of calorie intake) to prevent gains in body fat.

STEP 4: MONITOR YOUR PROGRESS

- Initial weight gains may be fairly rapid but you can expect to gain between ½–1 kg per month thereafter.
- Rapid gains in weight once you are on an established programme may indicate excess body fat gain.
- Keep a record of your body fat percentage, body weight and body measurements (vital statistics).

FIVE TIPS FOR GAINING WEIGHT

1 Do not skip meals or leave long gaps between eating.
2 Eat bigger portions than usual.
3 Eat high calorie foods, not high fat foods.
4 Supplement your food intake with liquid foods, such as milk-based drinks and fruit juice.
5 Add extra carbohydrate and protein to your meals, e.g. dried fruit, nuts, yoghurts, rather than extra fats, e.g. butter.

TEN ENERGY SNACKS FOR GAINING WEIGHT

1 Low fat Muffins (see pages 225–228).
2 Energy bars, cereal bars and fruit bars.
3 Home-made snack bars, e.g. Apricot Bars (see page 211), Fruit and Nut Bars (see page 211), and Muesli Bars (see page 209).
4 Dried fruit: raisins, sultanas, dates, apricots, peaches, figs, mango, papaya.
5 Fruit juice and smoothies.
6 Yoghurt and fromage frais.
7 Rolls and sandwiches filled with peanut butter, cheese, chicken, cottage cheese, tuna, ham, prawns, hummus or banana.
8 Milk and milkshakes.
9 Meal replacement supplements e.g. shakes and bars.
10 Nuts and seeds.

Protein and exercise

Regular exercisers need between 1.2–1.8 g protein/kg body weight per day, approximately twice as much as sedentary people (0.75 g/kg per day). This is equivalent to approximately 15% of your energy needs.

THREE REASONS WHY REGULAR EXERCISERS NEED MORE PROTEIN

1 Exercise increases the breakdown of muscle proteins into amino acids (catabolism) for use as fuel.
2 To repair tissue damage and maintain muscle mass.
3 To facilitate new muscle tissue growth.

HOW MUCH PROTEIN?

Athletes involved in strength and power activities, e.g. weight training, sprinting and bodybuilding need more protein than endurance athletes: 1.4–1.8 g/kg per day.

Athletes involved in aerobic activities, e.g. long distance running, aerobic classes and swimming need 1.2–1.4 g/kg per day.

Studies prove that a low protein diet will result in a loss of lean body mass. In other words, if you do not eat enough protein to meet your needs, muscle mass is lost and no new tissue growth occurs. Strength and body weight are therefore reduced.

On the other hand, a high protein diet is not beneficial either. Excessive protein is converted into a fuel source rather than lean tissue, and may be used for energy or stored as glycogen or fat. Eating more protein than you need will not result in additional strength or lean mass gains.

SUPPLEMENTS FOR WEIGHT GAIN			
	WHAT IS IT?	WHAT ARE THE BENEFITS?	SIDE EFFECTS?
Meal replacement supplement	Shake or bar providing whey protein, carbohydrate, vitamins, minerals and other nutrients	Increases nutritional intake, convenient and portable	None
Creatine	A protein (also made in the body) that combines with phosphate to make the high-energy compound, phosphocreatine	May increase strength and muscle mass, prolong maximal power output, and speed recovery between sets	Weight gain (as fluid and muscle mass). Strength gains may only be temporary
HMB	A derivative of the amino acid, leucine	May increase muscle mass and strength, improve recovery after exercise, reduce fat	None to date
Glutamine	An amino acid, abundant in muscle	Helps prevent excessive muscle breakdown during intense exercise; boosts immunity	None to date

BULKING UP EATING PLAN I

- This eating plan provides approximately 3000 kcal per day.
- In addition, you should include a minimum of 2 litres of fluid per day plus ½–1 litre for each hour of training. Each pre- and post-workout snack should be accompanied by 150–250 ml water.
- Where one portion of fruit is indicated on the menu, check page 3 for portion sizes.

Day 1	Breakfast	4 Weetabix or Shredded Wheat 450 ml (¾ pint) skimmed or semi-skimmed milk 50 g (2 oz) dried fruit I carton low fat yoghurt
	Snack	I sandwich: 2 thick slices of bread with 40 g (1½ oz) cheese and salad 2 portions fresh fruit
	Lunch	300 g (11 oz) jacket potato filled with 100 g (4 oz) tuna, chicken or turkey mixed with a little fromage frais Large mixed salad with I tbsp oil/vinegar dressing I carton low fat yoghurt I portion fresh fruit
	Pre-workout snack	2 bananas
	Post-workout snack	400 ml glucose polymer or energy drink
	Dinner	75 g (3 oz) pasta with Chicken and Mushroom Sauce (see page 157) Broccoli or other green vegetables Fruit Rice Pudding (see page 218)
Day 2	Breakfast	Milkshake: 250 ml (½ pint) semi-skimmed milk, I carton (150 g) low fat yoghurt, 225 g (8 oz) chopped fresh or tinned fruit (e.g. strawberries, peaches, bananas) 2 slices toast with honey
	Snack	I sandwich: 2 slices of bread with a little butter or low fat spread, I tbsp peanut butter and sliced tomatoes

	Lunch	2 Lean Hamburgers (see page 203) 2 portions fresh fruit
	Pre-workout snack	375 ml (⅔ pint) isotonic sports drink (home-made or commercial)
	Post-workout snack	3 slices malt loaf
	Dinner	175 g (6 oz) cod or haddock steak baked in foil with herbs and lemon juice I large (300 g/II oz) jacket potato with I tbsp plain yoghurt Peas and carrots Baked Bananas (see page 222) I carton (150 g) low fat yoghurt
Day 3	Breakfast	2 boiled/poached/scrambled eggs 3 slices wholemeal toast with a little butter/low fat spread
	Snack	Meal replacement shake or bar and I banana
	Lunch	Rice with Haddock and Peas (see page 136) Side salad with I tbsp oil/vinegar dressing 2 portions fresh fruit
	Pre-workout snack	2 Fruit and Nut Bars (see page 211)
	Post-workout snack	600 ml (I pint) isotonic sports drink (home-made or commercial)
	Dinner	100 g (4 oz) grilled skinless chicken or turkey breast Potato Salad (see page 185) Tomatoes or other salad vegetable 2 portions fresh fruit I carton (150 g) low fat fromage frais

BULKING UP EATING PLAN II

- This eating plan provides approximately 4000 kcal per day.
- In addition, you should include a minimum of 2 litres of fluid per day plus ½–1 litre for each hour of training. Each pre- and post-workout snack should be accompanied by 150–250 ml water.
- Where one portion of fruit is indicated on the menu, check page 3 for portion sizes.

Day 1	Breakfast	Power Porridge (see page 194)
	Snack	Peanut Bagel Melt (see page 198) 1 glass (200 ml) fruit juice
	Lunch	3 sandwiches: 6 slices of bread with a little butter/low fat spread, filled with 150 g (5 oz) chicken, ham or low fat cheese, salad vegetables and 2 tbsp reduced fat dressing 1 carton (200 g) cold rice dessert 1 portion fresh fruit
	Pre-workout snack	400 ml glucose polymer or energy drink
	Post-workout snack	3 Banana Muffins (see page 227)
	Dinner	Baked Macaroni Pie (see page 159) Broccoli or other green vegetables Yoghurt and Fruit Pudding (see page 223)
	Snack	50 g (2 oz) breakfast cereal 300 ml (½ pint) skimmed or semi-skimmed milk 50 g (2 oz) dried fruit
Day 2	Breakfast	Omelette made with 2 eggs and 2 egg whites 2 slices grilled lean bacon or 25 g (1 oz) cheese Tomatoes and mushrooms 2 slices toast with a little butter/low fat spread and jam
	Snack	2 bagels with 2 tbsp jam

	Lunch	3 pitta breads with 150 g (5 oz) chicken or tuna and salad vegetables with 2 tbsp oil/vinegar dressing 2 bananas 1 carton (150 g) whole milk yoghurt
	Pre-workout snack	600 ml (1 pint) isotonic sports drink (home-made or commercial)
	Post-workout snack	3 Fruit and Nut Bars (see page 211)
	Dinner	175 g/6 oz grilled cod or haddock steak Perfect Potato Pie (see page 181) Broccoli or other green vegetables 2 cartons (150 g) whole milk yoghurt
	Snack	2 slices toast 40 g (1½ oz) cheese
Day 3	Breakfast	6 Breakfast Pancakes (see page 192)
	Snack	1 large glass (250 ml/½ pint) skimmed or semi-skimmed milk 2 rolls with a little butter/low fat spread and 50 g (2 oz) ham or cottage cheese
	Lunch	300 g (11 oz) jacket potato with a little butter/low fat spread Spicy Bean Topping (see page 177) Side salad with 1 tbsp oil/vinegar dressing 2 portions fresh fruit
	Pre-workout snack	2 energy bars
	Post-workout snack	600 ml (1 pint) isotonic sports drink (home-made or commercial) 6 rice cakes with fruit spread or jam
	Dinner	Chicken and Broccoli Stir Fry (see page 139) 2 slices bread with a little butter/low fat spread 2 portions fresh fruit 1 carton (150 g) fromage frais
	Snack	Meal replacement shake or bar, 1 portion of fruit

6 LOSING WEIGHT

Most people would like to shed a few surplus pounds to improve their appearance, health or confidence. A low body fat level is an especially important goal for athletes if they want to be competitive, since excess fat hinders physical performance. However, it is important not to become obsessed with dieting or embark on faddy weight loss methods.

Guidelines for safe and effective fat loss

LOSE WEIGHT SLOWLY
Experts recommend losing weight at a rate between ½–1 kg (1–2 lb) per week. Any faster and you risk losing muscle and depleting your glycogen reserves. To lose ½ kg (1 lb) of fat you need to create an energy deficit of 3500 kcal. So, by eating 500 fewer calories per day you will lose ½ kg (1 lb) per week. Increasing your energy expenditure will increase weight loss further.

DON'T CUT CALORIES TOO MUCH
When you cut your calorie intake your resting metabolic rate (RMR) (see pages 48–9) automatically falls as your body goes into famine mode. This means you need fewer calories to maintain your weight. The more severe the calorie drop the greater the decrease in your RMR. This could be between 10–30%. The best strategy is to reduce your calorie intake by no more than 15% or 500 kcal per day and maintain or increase your activity level. Never eat less than your resting metabolic rate.

REDUCE YOUR FAT INTAKE
Aim to consume 15–20% of your calories from fat. This is not a no-fat diet – some fat is essential (see page 10) and can actually stop you feeling hungry. Make a food diary to identify the main sources of fat in your diet. Remember fat contains more calories (9 kcal/g) than carbohydrate or protein (4 kcal/g) so cutting down on high-fat foods quickly

reduces your calorie intake. Swap high fat foods for low fat nutritious alternatives (see below); replace high fat snacks with fresh fruit and vegetables and use less fat in your cooking.

EAT ENOUGH CARBOHYDRATE

Carbohydrates fuel all types of exercise and should continue to make up 60% of your calorie intake. If you eat too little carbohydrate you will experience fatigue, lack energy and your training will suffer. Low carbohydrate diets can result in muscle loss.

CHOOSE HIGH FIBRE, FILLING FOODS

High fibre foods fill you up, satisfy your appetite and keep hunger at bay. Base your meals and snacks on the following nutritious bulky foods:

- wholegrain breakfast cereals
- porridge
- wholemeal bread and pasta
- brown rice and other whole grains
- beans and lentils
- potatoes and starchy vegetables
- fresh fruit
- all kinds of vegetables.

EAT LITTLE AND OFTEN

Aim to eat 5–6 small meals or snacks per day at regular intervals. This will maintain energy levels, prevent hunger and avoid fat storage.

WHAT IS YOUR RESTING METABOLIC RATE?

Your resting metabolic rate (RMR) is the number of calories your body would burn if you did absolutely nothing but lie down for 24 hours a day. It is basically the energy used to keep your essential body functions ticking over and accounts for 60–75% of your total daily energy expenditure.

HOW MANY CALORIES DO YOU NEED PER DAY?
I Estimate your RMR

18–30 years   (weight (kg) $\times$ 14.7) + 496 = **RMR**
31–60 years   (weight (kg) $\times$ 8.7) + 829 = **RMR**

2 Estimate the number of calories you need for daily activities
Multiply your RMR by one of the numbers below according to your daily activity level.
Sedentary (mostly seated or standing activities) = RMR $\times$ 1.4
Moderately active (some walking during the day or active hobbies)
                                        = RMR $\times$ 1.7
Very active (physically active during the day)   = RMR $\times$ 2.0

3 Estimate the number of calories you burn during exercise
Estimate your weekly exercise energy expenditure, then divide by 7 to give a daily average value.

SPORT	KCAL PER HOUR
Aerobics (high intensity)	520
Aerobics (low intensity)	400
Badminton	370
Boxing (sparring)	865
Cycling (10 miles/h)	385
Cycling (5.5 miles/h)	250
Judo	760
Rowing machine	445
Running (6 mins/mile)	1000
Running (9 mins/mile)	750
Squash	615
Swimming (fast)	630
Tennis (singles)	415
Weight training	270–450

Figures are based on the calorie expenditure of an athlete weighing 65 kg. Values will be greater for heavier body weights; lower for smaller body weights.

4 Final step
Add together the figures for steps 2 and 3.

FAT-LOSS STRATEGIES

Increase your fat free mass. Regular weight training will significantly raise your RMR in as little as three months. One pound of muscle burns approximately 30–50 kcal per day per pound. So adding just one pound of muscle would use up an extra 350 kcal per week purely for maintenance purposes.

Regular aerobic workouts. Aerobic exercise can increase your RMR for between 6 and 36 hours after exercise. The greater the intensity of the workout and the longer the duration, the greater this effect will be.

Get more active. Exercise will compensate for some of the reduction in lean body mass that normally occurs during dieting and will, therefore, produce a smaller drop in the RMR.

SET POINT THEORY OF BODY WEIGHT

Researchers believe everyone has their own pre-determined 'set point', a weight or body fat range at which the body happily settles. This cannot easily be changed and is controlled by the interaction of several genes. If body fat levels increase, the metabolic rate increases and appetite decreases. Similarly, if body fat levels dip too low, the metabolic rate slows down and the appetite increases in an attempt to stabilise the body weight around the set point. That's why it is important to choose a realistic or attainable weight loss goal. (Some scientists argue that the set point can be reset over time by high intensity exercise and a low fat diet.)

LIFESTYLE FACTORS THAT MAKE YOU FAT

- No organised meal times
- Emotional/boredom eating
- Eating in front of the television/no social interaction
- Eating too fast
- Eating high fat foods

Setting personal goals

Make a commitment. Lose weight because you want to, not to please someone else. Your motivation must come from within. It helps to compile a list of reasons why you want to lose weight. Write down your goal and place it somewhere you will see it every day.

Establish your priorities. Before starting a weight loss programme, make sure you are not distracted by other problems, such as relationship or financial problems. These can take up a lot of mental and physical energy, setting you up for failure. If you are unhappy with other aspects of your life you are less likely to succeed with your programme.

Set a realistic goal. Try to achieve a comfortable weight you maintained earlier as a young adult. Don't set a goal that you have never achieved in your adult years or one which conforms to unrealistic social/fitness ideals. Set mini-targets, e.g. monthly weight loss goals.

Learn to recognise genuine hunger. Eat only when you are hungry, not for emotional reasons or through boredom. Do not deny hunger however, otherwise you will end up overeating later on. Learn to stop eating when you are satisfied.

CHANGING YOUR DIET

- Start your day with fruit, yoghurt, wholegrain cereal, porridge, wholemeal toast or low fat muffins.
- Include five portions of fruit and vegetables in your daily diet – eat fresh fruit as a snack, pile salad into your sandwich or add a side salad to your main meal.
- Make vegetables and grains the base of your meals – pasta, potatoes, rice, cous cous, bulgar wheat.
- Reduce saturated fats, e.g. butter, meat, pastry, biscuits, puddings.
- Avoid foods made with animal fats or hydrogenated vegetable fats as they contain larger amounts of trans fatty acids, e.g. margarine, biscuits, cakes and bakery items.
- Flavour salads and vegetables with herbs, lemon/lime juice, fruit vinegar.
- Add extra vegetables to pasta and curry sauces, stews, soups, bakes, shepherds pie, lasagne and moussaka.
- Make fresh fruit the base for dessert – add yoghurt, fromage frais, custard or half fat crème fraîche.

LOW FAT SNACKS

- Sandwiches/rolls/pitta/bagels (filled with cottage cheese, banana, salad, honey, marmite, tuna, chicken, turkey or ham)
- Low fat yoghurt and fromage frais
- Fresh fruit (e.g. apples, bananas, nectarines, grapes)
- English muffins/scones/crumpets/potato cakes
- Dried fruit
- Dried fruit bars/low fat energy bars/cereal bars
- Rice cakes/crackers/bread sticks

Low fat foods

Only eat low fat versions of foods if you like the taste. Don't expect low fat versions of foods to taste exactly the same as their high fat equivalents – they won't satisfy your taste expectations and you will end up eating the high fat version anyway. If you prefer genuine ice cream to the low fat/low calorie version, simply have a smaller portion. Accompany with your favourite fresh fruit to make a filling dessert.

Make sure you keep the portion sizes the same. If a low fat version contains half the fat of the ordinary food, that doesn't mean you can eat twice as much! For example, if you switch to a low fat salad dressing, don't use two tablespoons on your salad instead of one.

Substitute high fat cooking ingredients with low fat versions. For example, you may be better off using low fat foods such as skimmed milk and reduced fat cheese in cooking (e.g. sauces, custard, lasagne, macaroni cheese) where the taste difference is not too obvious.

Don't use low fat foods as an excuse to indulge in high fat treats. For example, if you eat diet yoghurt for dessert during the week, don't ruin your fat saving by indulging in creamy puddings at the weekend.

Low fat foods cannot satisfy strong cravings! If you crave a high fat food, allow yourself to eat a small portion once a week, rather than denying that craving and substituting low fat versions. For example, if you have a strong desire for a piece of chocolate, set aside one day a week to eat a small amount of your favourite brand. If you eat a reduced fat substitute, that may not satisfy your craving so you may end up bingeing on the real thing anyway.

Don't rely on ready meals. Most calorie counted ready meals are not very filling owing to their small portion size and low fat content. Fill the hunger gap by adding extra vegetables and follow with fresh fruit.

HOW TO CONTROL YOUR APPETITE NATURALLY

- Keep a food diary – identify situations and emotions that make you overeat.
- Ignore what the clock says – eat only when hungry, not just because it's one o'clock.
- Plan to eat at intervals of 2–4 hours rather than at specific times.
- Be more flexible with meal times – don't make rigid rules.
- Don't deny genuine hunger in an effort to hang on until meal times.
- If you find yourself wanting to eat out of boredom, plan enjoyable activities to fill in the gaps.
- Don't bury your emotions in food – deal with the problem in another way.
- Learn to leave food on the plate if you are full.
- Eat slowly – it takes 20 minutes for 'full-up' signals to reach the brain. Wait before eating second helpings.
- Ask: would I still want to eat this food if it wasn't there?

Exercise to burn fat

Exercise is the other half of the equation in weight loss. The best way to manage your weight permanently is to combine a programme of regular exercise with a balanced low fat diet.

CARDIOVASCULAR EXERCISE

How much?

The Health Development Agency and American College of Sports Medicine recommend 15–60 minutes of aerobic exercise 3–5 times per week. This need not necessarily occur in one continuous session but could be broken up into shorter sessions. For example, instead of spending 45 minutes on the stepping machine, you can take a 10-minute walk in the morning, a 20-minute swim at lunch time and 15 minutes' gardening in the evening.

High or low intensity?

Both high and low intensity exercise burns fat but you'll get faster results by exercising at an intensity that is around 85% of your maximum heart rate (220 minus your age). Although you will be burning a lower percentage of fat calories and a higher percentage of carbohydrate calories, you will be burning a lot more calories in total, and that means more fat in total. For example, walking burns around 270 kcal per hour, of which approx 60% (or 160 kcal) comes from fat. Running burns around 680 kcal, of which 40% (or 270 kcal) comes from fat. In other words, the more calories you burn the more fat you burn.

However, beginners should start with low-intensity activities as these are better suited to lower levels of fitness.

STRENGTH TRAINING

Strength training can help you lose fat faster because of its positive effect on your body composition and metabolic rate. As well as developing muscular strength, it helps develop and maintain lean body mass. The importance of lean mass (mainly muscle) is that it burns a significant number of calories just to exist – up to 50 kcal per day per pound – far more calories than fat. So if you increase your muscle mass by seven pounds, for example, you increase the number of calories your body burns throughout the day by 350 kcal.

Body image

Some athletes constantly strive to attain a very low weight or a different shape. They set themselves an unrealistic goal and believe that weight loss will help to solve their problems. Such individuals are usually highly self-disciplined perfectionists and very competitive. Unfortunately weight loss is not the solution. The problem is often one of a low self-esteem and a distorted body image. This can develop into a vicious circle of undereating, overeating and guilt.

HOW TO IMPROVE YOUR BODY IMAGE

- Learn to accept and like your body shape – it is unique to you – and try to emphasise your good points.
- Tell yourself that reducing your weight will not solve deep rooted problems or an emotional crisis.
- Practise seeing yourself in front of the mirror in a positive way.
- Stick to a low fat healthy diet in general but don't become obsessed by it.
- Eat whenever you are hungry – don't deny genuine hunger otherwise you will overeat later on and feel guilty.

- If you have overeaten, do not starve yourself later to punish yourself. Eat normally at your next meal.
- Make a list of your 'forbidden' foods. Make a point of eating a small amount of one of these each day for a week (e.g. one biscuit). You will find you won't gain weight and you won't feel guilty.
- Do not ban any foods – no food is suddenly going to make your weight balloon.
- Think of all food as a source of nutrients that will make our body healthier, not as a source of calories.
- Don't set yourself calorie goals. Learn to eat to your appetite.
- Enjoy eating with others – it is one of life's great pleasures.

WEIGHT LOSS EATING PLAN I

- The following eating plan is based on 1500 kcal per day.
- In addition to the foods listed, you should also include a minimum of 2 litres (4 pints) of fluid plus 1 litre (2 pints) for each hour of training. Each pre- and post-workout snack should be accompanied by 150–250 ml water.
- Where one portion of fruit is indicated, check page 3 for portion sizes.

Day I	Breakfast	I medium bowl (50 g/2 oz) wholegrain breakfast cereal 200 ml (⅓ pint) skimmed or semi-skimmed milk I portion fresh fruit
	Snack	4 rice cakes I banana
	Lunch	'Cream' of Tomato Soup (see page 114) I wholemeal roll with low fat spread Vegetable crudités (e.g. peppers, carrots, celery) I portion fresh fruit
	Pre-workout snack	50 g (2 oz) raisins
	Post-workout snack	I Raisin Muffin (see page 225)
	Dinner	I Fish Burger (see page 202) Large green salad with I tbsp Italian Dressing (see page 127) Yoghurt and Fruit Pudding (see page 223)

Day 2	Breakfast	2 slices wholemeal toast with low fat spread and Marmite I portion fresh fruit
	Snack	2 portions fresh fruit
	Lunch	2 slices wholemeal toast Half a large tin (210 g) baked beans I carton (150 g) very low fat fromage frais I portion fresh fruit
	Pre-workout snack	I Oaty Fruit Bar (see page 210)
	Post-workout snack	4 rice cakes
	Dinner	Quick Supper Salad (see page 122) I medium jacket potato (225 g/8 oz) with a little yoghurt or fromage frais, I portion fresh fruit, chopped and mixed with I carton (150 g) low calorie yoghurt
Day 3	Breakfast	I carton (150 g) low calorie yoghurt I portion fresh fruit I slice wholemeal toast with low fat spread and Marmite
	Snack	I Muesli Bar (see page 209) I portion fresh fruit
	Lunch	I wholemeal bap with 50 g (2 oz) chicken and salad Side salad with I tbsp reduced fat dressing 2 portions fresh fruit
	Pre-workout snack	I banana
	Post-workout snack	I Oatmeal Muffin (see page 227)
	Dinner	Quick Vegetable Curry (see page 137) 75 g (3 oz) rice (uncooked weight) I carton (150 g) low fat plain yoghurt with 100 g (4 oz) chopped fruit

WEIGHT LOSS EATING PLAN II

- The following eating plan is based on 1750 kcal per day.
- In addition to the foods listed, you should also include a minimum of 2 litres (4 pints) fluid plus 1 litre (2 pints) for each hour of training. Each pre- and post-workout snack should be accompanied by 150–250 ml water.
- Where one portion of fruit is indicated, check page 3 for portion sizes.

Day 1	Breakfast	1 glass (150 ml/5 fl oz) fruit juice 1 wholemeal English muffin with low fat spread and a little honey 1 glass (150 ml/5 fl oz) skimmed or semi-skimmed milk
	Snack	2 portions fresh fruit
	Lunch	Brown Rice and Bean Salad (see page 124) Vegetable crudités (e.g. peppers, carrots, celery) 1 portion fresh fruit 1 carton (150 g) low calorie yoghurt
	Pre-workout snack	1 large banana
	Post-workout snack	1 slice Banana Cake (see page 229)
	Dinner	Vegetable Gratin with Potatoes (see page 184) Hot Winter Fruit Salad or Cool Summer Fruit Salad (see page 219)
Day 2	Breakfast	2 slices wholemeal toast with low fat spread and a little honey or fruit spread 1 portion fresh fruit 1 carton (150 g) low calorie yoghurt
	Snack	1 portion fresh fruit 1 Raisin Scone (see page 212)

	Lunch	Turkey Pockets (see page 198) Large green salad with 1 tbsp Italian Dressing (see page 127) 1 portion fresh fruit
	Pre-workout snack	300 ml isotonic sports drink (home-made or commercial)
	Post-workout snack	50 g (2 oz) dried fruit
	Dinner	Mexican Bean Bake (see page 146) 1 medium jacket potato (225 g/8 oz) with a little yoghurt or fromage frais 1 portion fresh fruit 150 ml (¼ pint) low fat custard
Day 3	Breakfast	1 medium bowl (50 g/2 oz) wholegrain breakfast cereal 200 ml (⅓ pint) skimmed or semi-skimmed milk 1 portion fresh fruit
	Snack	1 carton (150 g) low calorie yoghurt 1 thick slice toast with low fat spread and Marmite
	Lunch	1 wholemeal pitta with salad and 60 g (2 oz) sliced turkey, chicken or ham Side salad with 1 tbsp reduced fat dressing 2 portions fresh fruit
	Pre-workout snack	1 cereal bar
	Post-workout snack	3 Oatmeal Cookies (see page 213)
	Dinner	75 g (3 oz) pasta (uncooked weight) A–Z Vegetable Sauce (see page 154) topped with 50 g (2 oz) low fat soft cheese or fromage frais 1 carton (150 g) low fat plain yoghurt with 100 g (4 oz) chopped fruit

THE VEGETARIAN ATHLETE

A couple of decades ago, the traditional 'meat and two veg' was regarded as the mainstay of an athlete's diet. Now more and more athletes are shunning meat in favour of a different style of eating. Meat-free diets range from a strict vegan diet to a more relaxed pescatarian diet (includes fish). These can be equally – if not more – healthy for active people, owing partly to the high carbohydrate/low fat content and partly to the higher content of fresh fruit and vegetables.

Current thinking is that a meat-free diet can provide athletes with all the essential nutrients needed by the body. But before embarking on a new style of eating, whether for health or ethical reasons, you need to know the pitfalls as well as the benefits.

Vegan diet (excludes meat, poultry, fish, dairy products and eggs)

Benefits. Vegans tend to be leaner and lighter than the rest of the population and obesity is less common. This is mainly due to their lower caloric and fat intake. The strong emphasis on fruit, pulses and vegetables means you get plenty of fibre, vitamins, minerals, unsaturated fats and phytochemicals (plant substances with cancer-fighting properties).

Pitfalls. Vegans may have low intakes of protein, calcium, iron, vitamin B_{12}, vitamin D and iodine. Dairy products are a major source of calcium so make sure you eat alternative calcium sources (see overleaf). You may be at risk of pernicious anaemia unless you include vitamin B_{12}, found in fortified foods such as soya milk, tofu, breakfast cereals, yeast extract, vegetable stocks, soya burger mixes, or a supplement. Recommended supplements: vitamin B_{12} (in a multivitamin or B complex); calcium (with vitamin D or in a multivitamin/mineral).

FOOD CONTAINING 250 mg CALCIUM
(APPROX. ⅓ RDA)

- 50 g (2 oz) tofu
- 100 g (4 oz) hummus
- 2 tbsp sunflower or sesame seeds
- 350 g (12 oz) cooked beans
- 7 slices white bread
- 5 figs
- 10 tbsp spinach or spring cabbage
- 4 oranges

Vegetarian diet (excludes meat and fish)

Benefits. Vegetarians are 40% less likely to develop cancer (especially of the breast, colon and prostate), and 30% less likely to suffer from heart disease. This is partly due to their healthier lifestyle and partly due to their diet which is lower in saturated fats and high in fibre, fruit and vegetables. The result is lower levels of blood cholesterol (especially the LDL (bad) cholesterol) and higher intakes of cancer-protective antioxidants.

Pitfalls. Omitting meat may result in lower intakes of iron and zinc and increased risk of iron-deficiency anaemia. The absorption of these minerals is reduced by plant substances such as fibre, phytates and oxalic acid. However, there is evidence that the body adapts over time by increasing the efficiency of iron and zinc absorption, so in reality the risk of iron-deficiency anaemia is small for long term vegetarians. Eating vitamin-C rich foods also greatly increases iron absorption and may counteract any negative effects of phytates. Zinc can be obtained from wholemeal bread, nuts, seeds and eggs.

Both vegetarians and vegans may go short of omega-3 fatty acids found in oily fish. Non-fish sources include soya bean and rapeseed oil, linseeds, walnuts, sweet potatoes, pumpkin seeds and omega-3 enriched eggs.

FOOD CONTAINING 3 mg IRON (⅕ FEMALE RDA; ⅓ MALE RDA)

- 2 tbsp (15 g) bran flakes
- Half a tin (240 g) baked beans
- 4 slices wholemeal bread
- 12 prunes
- 45 g (1½ oz) cashew nuts
- 150 g broccoli

Pescatarian diet (excludes meat and poultry; includes fish)

Benefits. Pescatarian diets are usually low in fat so, again, there's a lower risk of obesity and heart disease. Omega-3 fatty acids (providing oily fish varieties are eaten regularly) will be in good supply and this helps protect against strokes, thrombosis and heart attacks.

Pitfalls. Like vegetarians, the main nutrient likely to be in short supply is iron so you need to eat iron-rich plant foods (see page 64).

Omega-3 fatty acids may pose a problem if you stick only to white fish; include oily fish such as mackerel, sardines or herring in your diet once a week to get your recommended intake of these fatty acids.

Demi-vegetarian diet (excludes meat; includes poultry and fish)

Benefits. Typically lower in fat compared with diets containing meat, which will have a beneficial effect on blood cholesterol levels. It is easier to get all the vitamins and minerals from a demi-vegetarian diet than a vegetarian diet as it doesn't require a drastic change in eating habits.

Pitfalls. You may go short on iron if you eat only the light meat of poultry rather than the dark meat, e.g. a leg portion, which is relatively rich in iron. There is practically no iron in the light meat (breast) so eat both types of poultry meat to boost iron intake.

Chicken and turkey contain a good deal of fat in and beneath the skin, so ensure that you skin chicken or turkey portions before eating.

Getting enough protein

Protein is found in a wide variety of plant foods, including cereals, pulses, nuts, seeds and soya products, as well as dairy products and eggs. Vegetarians eating a variety of these foods each day will be consuming a mixture of proteins that complement each other. Any shortfall of amino acids in one protein source can be compensated for by greater amounts in another source, thus increasing the overall biological value (or usefulness) of the proteins. For example, cereals are low in lysine and rich in methionine. These are complemented by pulses which are rich in lysine and low in methionine. So, beans on toast or lentils with rice would make excellent meals.

The proteins in foods from the following categories complement each other. Plan your meals to incude two or more categories:

1 *Pulses* – beans, lentils, peas
2 *Grains* – bread, pasta, rice, oats, breakfast cereals
3 *Nuts and seeds* – peanuts, peanut butter, almonds, cashews, sunflower seeds, pumpkin seeds
4 *Quorn* – Quorn mince, fillets and burgers
5 *Soya* – tofu, soya mince, burgers and sausages, soya milk, soya 'yoghurt'
6 *Dairy* – milk, cheese, yoghurt

Suitable protein combinations include:

- Pasta with lentil bolognese
- Porridge made with milk
- Tofu and vegetable stirfry with rice
- Quorn burger with a bap
- Peanut butter sandwich

Is it a healthier diet?

Scientific studies of vegetarians have found that, in general, they live longer and are healthier than people who eat meat. They suffer much less from illnesses such as cancer, heart disease, high blood pressure and other common health problems. The 12-year Oxford Health Study (1994) of more than 6000 vegetarians and 5000 meat-eaters found that vegetarians had a 30% lower risk of heart disease, a 40% lower risk of cancer (especially breast and colon), and were 20% less likely to die of any specific cause. They also had a lower risk of bowel disorders, diabetes and osteoporosis.

TOP TIPS FOR GOING VEGETARIAN

- Cut back on meat gradually and introduce more pulses, e.g. beans, lentils, chick peas, in your diet.
- Include more grains and cereals, e.g. bread, barley, oats, buckwheat, cous cous.
- Choose low fat versions of dairy products.
- Try adding different types of nuts and seeds to food, e.g. vegetables and almond stir fry; vegetable/bean curry with cashews; sunflower or sesame seeds in home-made cakes; peanut burgers.
- Buy some good vegetarian cookery books.
- Don't always eat cheese/eggs in place of meat.
- If you are not used to a high fibre diet, use a mixture of wholemeal/white cereal products to start with. Increase fibre-rich foods gradually.

Easy menu planner

Plan your vegetarian diet around the following four main food groups to ensure you get the right balance of amino acids and all the nutrients needed for good health.

FRUIT AND VEGETABLES 5+ servings/day	LEGUMES AND VEGETARIAN PROTEIN FOOD 2–3 servings/day or 4–5 if dairy excluded
Vegetables and fruit are packed with vitamin C, beta-carotene, iron, calcium and fibre. Try to eat at least one serving of a dark green leafy vegetable (e.g. broccoli, spinach) and one serving of yellow/orange vegetables or fruit (e.g. carrots, tomatoes) each day.	Beans, lentils and peas are good sources of protein, fibre, iron, calcium, zinc and B vitamins. This group also includes eggs, nuts, seeds, soya milk (fortified), soya mince, tofu, tempeh, all of which supply protein, vitamins and minerals.
Serving size = 1 apple/pear/ orange; 100 g (4 oz) any fruit or vegetables; 3 heaped tbsp cooked vegetables; 2 carrots.	**Serving size** = 100 g (4 oz) cooked pulses, tofu, soya mince; 2 eggs; 25 g (1 oz) nuts or seeds.

CEREALS AND STARCHY VEGETABLES 5–11 servings/day depending on activity level	MILK AND DAIRY PRODUCTS 2–3 servings/day
This group includes bread, rice pasta, breakfast cereals and potatoes. They are rich in complex carbohydrates as well as B vitamins and certain minerals.	This group includes milk, yoghurt and cheese. Choose the low fat versions wherever possible. They supply calcium, protein and B vitamins.
Serving size = 1 slice of bread; 25 g (1 oz) uncooked grains or breakfast cereal; 75 g (3 oz) potato.	**Serving size** = 200 ml (⅓ pint) milk; 1 carton yoghurt/fromage frais; 40 g (1½ oz) hard cheese; 100 g (4 oz) cottage cheese.

Meeting your nutritional needs on a vegetarian diet

NUTRIENT	VEGETARIAN SOURCES
Protein	Milk, cheese, yoghurt, eggs, beans, lentils, peas, nuts, seeds, soya products, quorn.
Iron	Wholemeal bread, whole grains, nuts, pulses, green vegetables (e.g. broccoli, iron, watercress), fortified soya products, fortified breakfast cereals, seeds, dried fruit.
Vitamin B_{12}	Dairy products, eggs, fortified foods (e.g. soya products, breakfast cereals, yeast extract), soya burger mixes.
Calcium	Dairy products, sunflower and sesame seeds, spinach, broccoli, almonds, brazils, fortified soya products (e.g. tofu, figs).
Zinc	Whole grains, wholemeal bread, pulses, nuts, seeds, eggs.
Iodine	Seaweed, iodised salt.

VEGETARIAN ATHLETE'S EATING PLAN

- The following six-day menu provides approximately 2500 kcal per day. Decrease or increase the quantities according to your individual calorie requirements (see page 49).
- In addition to the foods listed, you should also include a minimum of 2 litres (4 pints) of fluid plus 1 litre (2 pints) for each hour of training. Each pre- and post-workout snack should be accompanied by 150–250 ml water.
- Where one portion of fruit is indicated, check page 3 for portion sizes.

Day 1	Breakfast	1 large bowl (75 g/3 oz) wholegrain breakfast cereal 200 ml (⅓ pint) skimmed or semi-skimmed milk 1 portion fresh fruit
	Snack	1 Date and Walnut Bar (see page 210) 1 portion fresh fruit
	Lunch	Athlete's Cold Pasta Salad with red kidney beans (see page 121) 1 portion fresh fruit 1 carton (150 g) low fat yoghurt
	Pre-workout snack	50 g (2 oz) raisins or dates
	Post-workout snack	2 Oatmeal Muffins (see page 227)
	Dinner	300 g (11 oz) jacket potato 100 g (4 oz) fromage frais/cottage cheese Large green salad with 1 tbsp Italian Dressing (see page 127) 2 Oatmeal and Raisin Scotch Pancakes (see page 224) 1 portion fresh fruit
Day 2	Breakfast	Raisin Toast (see page 168) 1 glass (200 ml) fruit juice
	Snack	25 g (1 oz) nuts (e.g. cashews, almonds) 25 g (1 oz) raisins
	Lunch	2 thick slices wholemeal toast with butter/low fat spread

		Half a large tin (210 g) baked beans Side salad 1 carton (150 g) low fat fromage frais 1 portion fresh fruit
	Pre-workout snack	1 large banana
	Post-workout snack	4 rice cakes with 4 heaped tsp fruit spread
	Dinner	Spicy Bean Enchiladas (see page 143) 1 medium (225 g/8 oz) jacket potato with a little butter/low fat spread Broccoli or carrots Low Fat Tiramisu (see page 222)
Day 3	Breakfast	1 egg (boiled/poached/scrambled) 2 thick slices wholemeal toast with butter/low fat spread and Marmite 1 portion fresh fruit
	Snack	1 wholemeal English muffin with fruit spread or honey 1 portion fresh fruit
	Lunch	Millet Pilaff with Nuts and Raisins (see page 142) Side salad with 1 tbsp reduced fat dressing 2 portions fresh fruit
	Pre-workout snack	1 fruit bar
	Post-workout snack	1 banana sandwich (2 slices wholemeal bread and 1 sliced banana)
	Dinner	Bean and Tomato Casserole (see page 145) 75 g (3 oz) rice (uncooked weight) Broccoli or other green vegetables 1 carton (150 g) low fat plain yoghurt with 1 tbsp granola-type cereal
Day 4	Breakfast	3 Breakfast Muffins (see page 191) 1 portion fresh fruit
	Snack	1 carton (150 g) low fat yoghurt 1 portion fresh fruit
	Lunch	Greek Filled Pitta (see page 199) 2 portions fresh fruit

	Pre-workout snack	I energy bar
	Post-workout snack	2 Banana Muffins (see page 227)
	Dinner	Store-cupboard Bean Bake (see page 144) 75 g (3 oz) pasta (uncooked weight) Mixed salad with I tbsp oil/vinegar dressing 100 g (4 oz) tinned apricots 150 ml (¼ pint) low fat custard
Day 5	Breakfast	75 g (3 oz) muesli (no added sugar) 150 ml (¼ pint) skimmed or semi-skimmed milk I carton (150 g) low fat yoghurt
	Snack	2 slices Banana Bread (see page 171) or Blueberry Bread (see page 172)
	Lunch	2 sandwiches: 4 slices wholemeal bread with low fat soft cheese, dates and chopped walnuts Vegetable crudités (e.g. carrots, celery, red peppers) 2 portions fresh fruit
	Pre-workout snack	2 slices toast with fruit spread or jam
	Post-workout snack	I banana 4 rice cakes
	Dinner	75 g (3 oz) pasta Vegetarian Chilli Sauce (see page 154) Large side salad with I tbsp Italian dressing (see page 127) 2 portions fresh fruit
Day 6	Breakfast	2 Breakfast Pancakes (see page 192) I glass (200 ml) fruit juice
	Snack	I wholemeal roll filled with 50 g (2 oz) cottage cheese
	Lunch	2 Muffin Pizzas (see page 200) Large side salad with I tbsp oil/vinegar dressing
	Pre-workout snack	2 Fruit Buns (see page 173)

	Post-workout snack	4 low fat crackers 1 portion fresh fruit
	Dinner	Dahl (see page 145) 75 g (3 oz) rice (uncooked weight) Broccoli or other green vegetables Hot Winter Fruit Salad or Cool Summer Fruit Salad (see page 219)
Day 7	Breakfast	Bagel, toasted and topped with cottage cheese and pineapple 1 portion fresh fruit
	Snack	2 portions fresh fruit
	Lunch	Lentil and Vegetable Soup (see page 117) 2 wholemeal rolls with butter/low fat spread 2 portions fresh fruit
	Pre-workout snack	50 g (2 oz) dried fruit
	Post-workout snack	2 Apricot Bars (see page 211)
	Dinner	Vegetable Cous Cous (see page 140) Crunchy Apple Crumble (see page 218) 2 tbsp low fat yoghurt

8 EATING ON THE RUN

It's often difficult to squeeze healthy meals into a busy schedule. However, skipped meals, irregular meal times and hurried fatty snacks will leave you low in energy, glycogen and important vitamins and minerals. The following practical advice will help you develop healthy eating strategies that fit in with your hectic lifestyle.

Strategies for eating on the run

Organisation. Take your food with you so you won't end up skipping meals or grabbing the nearest high fat snack when you are ravenous.

Planning. Plan your day in advance so you always make time to eat no matter how busy your schedule is.

Identifying eating opportunities. Make a list of times and places where you could eat, e.g. in the changing room; sports club; killing time between appointments; driving or travelling; working at your desk.

Preparing ahead. Prepare meals in advance by cooking larger quantities one day and keeping the remainder in the fridge or freezer.

Shopping wisely. Routinely shop with a planned shopping list; this will save you a good deal of time and ensure you have enough food to last you for a week. Avoid frequent small shopping trips which cost you more time.

Stocking up. Keep healthy staple foods in your kitchen cupboard so you always have a good choice of healthy food to hand.

Eating healthily on the run

- Include at least one fruit or vegetables portion with each meal.
- If you must have chips and fried food for lunch, balance it out with a side salad and follow it with fresh fruit.
- Get into the breakfast habit every day – if you can't eat at home, take a healthy snack with you (see 'Healthy snacks' on p. 74).
- In restaurants, eat bigger portions of carbohydrate foods, e.g. pasta, bread or potatoes, and cut back on the rich sauces and puddings.
- Take healthy snacks like apples, satsumas, bananas or dried fruit with you.
- Choose speedy meals which contain less fat and more carbohydrates and vegetables, e.g. home-made vegetable soup (make a big pot in advance) and rolls, jacket potatoes with tuna or cottage cheese.
- Add a portion of salad (ready bought if you like) to your lunch time sandwiches.
- Drink at least 2 litres (4 pints) of fluid per day (allow an extra 1 litre (2 pints) for each hour of sport you play), e.g. water, diluted fruit juice, diluted squash or isotonic sports drinks.

Super sandwiches

Sandwiches make a high carbohydrate healthy meal for eating on the run. Ready prepared sandwiches from supermarkets and snack bars often contain butter and mayonnaise so check the label. A typical prawn mayonnaise sandwich can contain more than 22 g fat!

For a really healthy sandwich it is best to make your own. Cut thick slices of bread and choose one of the low fat fillings suggested below.

- Wholemeal bread with low fat soft cheese, dates and chopped walnuts.
- French baguette with tuna, tomato, watercress and low fat salad dressing.
- Malted grain bread with turkey or chicken and low calorie coleslaw.
- Ciabatta with reduced fat mozzarella, beef tomatoes, olives and low calorie salad dressing.
- Bap with chicken, dried apricots, celery and tarragon.

- Foccacia bread (cut into wedges) with roasted peppers, aubergine and onion.
- Pitta bread with crumbled feta, beansprouts, baby spinach and cucumber.
- Rye bread with cottage cheese and chopped dates.
- Wrap filled with sliced chicken, salad and taco relish.
- Rolls with ham, lettuce, grated carrot and low fat salad dressing.
- Olive bread with hummus and salad leaves.
- Raisin bread with banana, sultanas and cinnamon.
- Soda bread with mature grated Cheddar, tomato and lettuce.
- Bagel with low fat soft cheese, salmon and tomato.

SANDWICH FACT FILE

- Wholemeal bread contains twice as much fibre as white bread (6.5 g per 100 g compared with 2.8 g per 100 g).
- A thin spreading of butter equals about 5 g butter (4.1 g fat) per slice; a medium spreading is 7 g (5.7 g fat) and thickly spread it is 12 g (9.8 g fat).
- For a substantial meal, make a sandwich using three slices of bread.
- Mayonnaise contains 22 g fat per spoonful. Use fromage frais or low calorie salad dressing instead.
- If preparing sandwiches in advance, wrap and store in the fridge or an insulated cool bag.

EATING OUT GUIDE		
TYPE OF RESTAURANT	BEST CHOICES	WORST CHOICES
Indian	Chapatti, plain naan Chicken tikka Tandoori dishes Chickpea dishes (e.g. Channa Dahl) Lentil dishes (e.g. Dahl) Dry vegetable curries Vegetable side dishes	Samosas Anything fried Most meat curries and biryanis Anything in a korma, pasanda or masala sauce Roghan Josh
Chinese	Soup Vegetable, chicken or prawn chop suey Sweet and sour vegetables Stir-fried vegetables Rice and noodles	Peking duck Sweet and sour pork Spare ribs Prawn crackers Fried noodles
Pizza/Italian	Pasta with tomato/vegetable/seafood based sauces Pasta filled with spinach/ricotta Gnocchi with tomato-based sauce Pizza with vegetable toppings Salads: tomatoes, avocado, olives Vegetable risottos	Pasta with creamy/buttery sauces Pasta with Bolognese sauce Lasagne (meat) Pizza with meat, pepperoni, salami or extra cheese toppings Garlic bread, dough sticks
Fast food	Plain grilled hamburger Flame grilled chicken Salad Milkshake	Large/quarterpounder hamburgers Chicken burgers Chips/fries Anything fried Doughnuts Apple pies

TYPE OF RESTAURANT	BEST CHOICES	WORST CHOICES
Greek	Greek salad Tomato or cucumber salad Tzatziki and pitta bread Hummus Grilled fish Dolmades Stuffed tomatoes Fresh fruit	Moussaka Taramasalata Lamb dishes Keftethakia (meat balls) Baklava
French	Consommé Ratatouille Salads (e.g. Nicoise) Vegetable dishes Grilled chicken or fish	Anything in a creamy or buttery sauce Pastry dishes
Mexican	Guacamole Bean burritos, tortillas Vegetable fajitas Tostadas with beans or vegetables Vegetable chilli	Tortilla chips Potato skins Beef chilli Tortillas/burritos with meat Chimichangas

Store-cupboard stand-bys

Keep a basic stock of the following non-perishable foods in your store-cupboard so you've always got something healthy on stand-by for a quick meal.

TINS	PACKETS	JARS
Tomatoes Baked beans Various beans (e.g. red kidney, butter beans) Soup Fish (e.g. tuna, sardines) Rice pudding (low fat) Custard (low fat) Fruit in juice (e.g. pineapple, peaches)	Pasta Rice Other grains (e.g. cous cous, bulgar wheat, millet) Breakfast cereal Porridge oats Dried fruit (e.g. raisins, apricots, dates)	Pasta sauce Curry sauce Low fat cooking sauce Salsa Passata Honey, fruit spread, jam Dried herbs

Time-saving kitchen strategies

- Get all the ingredients together before you begin cooking.
- Cook as many ingredients as possible together in one saucepan by working backwards with the cooking times, e.g. add the chopped vegetables to the rice saucepan 10 minutes before the end of the rice cooking time; add tinned beans or tuna 5 minutes before the end.
- Make one huge bowl of mixed salad instead of several separate bowls of individual ingredients.
- Stir pasta sauces into the drained pasta and continue heating in the saucepan rather than heating the sauce in a separate pan.
- Multi-task – toss a salad or stir fry some vegetables while the potatoes are cooking in the microwave.
- Make one-pot meals.
- Make larger quantities than you need and save the remainder in the fridge or freezer.
- Use baking dishes or cooking dishes that double up as serving dishes.
- Organise your time efficiently, e.g. pop a couple of potatoes in the oven before you go for a workout; they will be ready by the time you return.

Healthy snacks

FOR TRAVELLING

The following snacks can be taken with you and eaten when travelling to competitions, in-between business appointments, in fact anytime you are on the move. They can all be prepared the day before and wrapped and packed into your kit bag or travelling case.

- Sandwiches, bagels, rolls and English muffins
- Fresh fruit
- Vegetable crudités, e.g. carrots, celery, peppers
- Home-made bread and cake (see pages 165–73 and 229–34)
- Fruit bars, cereal bars, energy bars, protein bars
- Home-made bars (see pages 209–23)
- Home-made muffins (see pages 225–8)
- Malt loaf
- Raisin bread
- Low fat yoghurt, cottage cheese and fromage frais
- Foil-wrapped chicken or turkey breast

- Mini pancakes
- Yoghurt drinks
- Meal replacement shakes (ready-to-drink cans)

FOR YOUR DESK DRAWER

Keep a supply of healthy non-perishable snacks in your desk drawer or briefcase so you can refuel while at work.

- Low fat crackers
- Breadsticks
- Rice cakes
- Dried fruit (apples, apricots, dates, raisins etc.)
- Long life fruit juice
- Tinned fruit (ring pull tins)
- Oatcakes
- Plain popcorn
- Mini boxes of breakfast cereals
- Fig rolls and low fat biscuits

SNACK SWAPS	
SNACK	HEALTHIER SNACK
Crisps	Plain popcorn
Tortilla chips	Breadsticks
Digestive biscuits	Rice cakes
Chocolate biscuits	Oatcakes
Chocolate bar	Fruit bar
Doughnut	Currant bun
Sweets	Raisins
Dairy ice cream	Low fat yoghurt
Slice of cake	Banana

Travelling overseas

When travelling overseas it is essential to plan your food intake. Local foods may turn out to be unsuitable for athletes or, in many cases, simply unavailable. One of the dangers of overseas travel is consuming contaminated food or drink and suffering from gastroenteritis (traveller's diarrhoea). Follow the guidelines below to ensure that you remain healthy while abroad.

- Research the types of foods likely to be available at your destination. Check the provision of local shops, your hotel/accommodation facility and the sports venue before you travel.
- Take a supply of non-perishable foods such as boxes of breakfast cereal, energy bars, fruit bars, rice cakes and crackers.
- Stick to plain and familiar foods. Do not experiment with unusual or spicy local delicacies.
- Drink only bottled water/drinks; avoid ice in drinks.
- Avoid unpasteurised milk and dairy products.
- Peel fruit and vegetables; avoid salads which may have been washed in tap water.
- Avoid dishes which are lukewarm or seem reheated.
- Avoid food sold from street vendors.
- Avoid fish and chicken dishes as far as possible unless they are piping hot, as there is a greater chance of contamination.

9 DRINKING

Exercise increases the production of heat from your body; sweating helps to keep you cool and stops you overheating. But fluid losses during exercise can be high (1–2 litres per hour in warm conditions) and it is easy to become dehydrated. If dehydration does set in, body temperature rises, performance suffers and heat stress results. Just a 2% reduction in body weight through dehydration causes a 10–20% loss of performance, early fatigue and circulatory stress. Higher losses cause nausea, dizziness, vomiting and, ultimately, heat stroke.

Early warning symptoms of heat stress

- Dizziness
- Fatigue
- Headache
- Feeling excessively hot
- Nausea
- Little or no sweating
- Cool skin
- Disorientation
- Confusion

Preventing dehydration

BEFORE EXERCISE

Ensure you are fully hydrated before exercise, then top up with around 200–250 ml (⅓–½ pint) of fluid 15–20 minutes beforehand. You can check for dehydration by noting the frequency, colour and volume of your urine. Aim for:

- light coloured urine
- high volume
- high frequency.

DURING EXERCISE
During exercise, regular drinking will help offset fluid losses and prevent dehydration. It is better to drink frequent small amounts than too much too quickly. If you feel thirsty you may already be dehydrated. Fluid empties more slowly from the stomach when you are dehydrated so this can make you feel nauseous and even cause vomiting, delaying fluid absorption even further. Aim to:

- consume 150–250 ml (¼–½ pint) water or isotonic drink every 10–20 minutes
- start drinking early; do not wait until you are thirsty
- consume 25–50 g (1–2 oz) carbohydrate per hour during strenuous exercise lasting more than 90 minutes.

POST-EXERCISE
It is important to replace fluid as rapidly as possible after exercise. Drink freely but do not stop once your thirst has been satisfied; you could still be dehydrated.

How much fluid?

This depends on how hard and long you have been exercising, the surrounding temperature and humidity, and also on your individual body chemistry. To get an idea of your fluid requirements, weigh yourself before and after exercise. The amount of weight lost corresponds to the amount of water lost as sweat – 1 kg is equivalent to 1 litre of water. For example, a weight loss of 1½ kg means you have lost 1½ litres of fluid. Aim to replace this amount plus more during and after exercise, allowing 1½ litres for each 1 litre of lost fluid, since you continue to sweat after exercise and urination increases after exercise. Your body weight should be fully restored within 3–4 hours of exercise.

What to drink?

If you are exercising for less than one hour at a low or moderate intensity, drinking plain (or flavoured unsweetened) water is fine. For longer or particularly strenuous workouts, sports drinks have a number of advantages.

BENEFITS OF A FLUID REPLACEMENT SPORTS DRINK

- More rapid replacement of fluid. The carbohydrate (sugars) speeds water absorption in the small intestine.
- Maintains blood volume and decreases urine output (due to sugar and sodium content). This is especially important during prolonged events, e.g. marathon, ultra-distance, cycle touring.
- Provides additional fuel. The sugars and glucose polymers in the drink provide readily available fuel which helps offset glycogen depletion and delays fatigue. Aim to consume 30–60 g per hour in events lasting more than 90 minutes. You can achieve this by drinking 1 litre of a drink containing 30–60 g carbohydrate.
- Pleasant taste. The drink must be palatable to encourage you to drink enough.

What to look for on the label of an isotonic sports drink

Types of carbohydrate

- Mostly glucose (dextrose) and sucrose; small amounts of glucose polymers or fructose are acceptable.
- Avoid high-fructose drinks.

Carbohydrate content

- 4–8 g/100 ml (isotonic)

Sodium content

- 40–110 mg/100 ml

Additives

You may wish to avoud products containing preservatives, artificial sweetners, colours and flavours. The best alternative is to make your own drink from pure fruit juice and water (see page 82).

GLOSSARY OF TERMS

Hypotonic
- A hypotonic drink is more dilute than body fluids, therefore it contains a lower concentration of particles (sugars and electrolytes) per 100 ml.
- Typical carbohydrate content: < 4 g/100 ml.
- Examples: water, low calorie or 'diet' drinks, very dilute squash, low calorie sports drinks.

Isotonic
- An isotonic drink contains the same concentration of particles (sugars and electrolytes) as body fluids and is absorbed in the small intestine faster than plain water.
- Typical carbohydrate content: 4–8 g/100 ml.
- Examples: diluted squash (1:4), diluted fruit juice (1:1), commercial isotonic sports drinks.

Energy drinks
- Energy drinks have a relatively high carbohydrate concentration (greater than that of body fluids), and usually contain no sodium. They are emptied more slowly from the stomach and absorbed more slowly than plain water.
- Typical carbohydrate concentration: 8–20 g/100 ml.

Glucose polymers/ malto-dextrins
- Glucose polymers are a common ingredient in sports drinks. They are made from chemically-treated corn-starch which breaks down to produce short chains of glucose molecules (4–20 units). They are closer to simple carbohydrates (sugars) than complex carbohydrates.
- The main advantage of adding them to sports drinks is that they increase the carbohydrate content of the drink (by 4–20 times depending on chain length) without affecting its osmolality ('concentration') and speed of absorption. In other words, they provide more carbohydrate per 100 ml than glucose or sucrose at the same 'concentration'. This is particularly useful for refuelling during strenuous events lasting for more than 90 minutes. Also, glucose polymers are not sweet tasting so a manufacturer can achieve a palatable drink with a high carbohydrate content by using a mixture of simple sugars and glucose polymers.

RULES OF THUMB

- If you are exercising for 30 minutes or less, water is a good fluid replacer.
- If you are exercising at a moderate intensity for up to 90 minutes, drink water or a hypotonic or isotonic drink.
- If you are exercising at a high intensity for up to 90 minutes, drink an isotonic sports drink.
- If you are exercising at a moderate or high intensity for longer than 90 minutes, drink an isotonic drink based on glucose polymers to provide extra fuel.

EIGHT WAYS TO KEEP COOL

1 Drink a minimum of two litres of fluid per day: water, diluted fruit juice and soft drinks, fruit or herb teas, weak tea.
2 Consume at least 150–250 ml (¼–½ pint) fluid for every 20–30 minutes of exercise.
3 Increase your fluid intake 24 hours prior to competition.
4 Drink more fluid during hot or humid weather.
5 Gradually acclimatise yourself to new weather conditions (allow up to two weeks).
6 Wear loose fitting natural fibre clothing during training that allows you to sweat freely and allows moisture to evaporate.
7 Practise your fluid replacement strategy during training, don't leave it until competition.
8 Experiment to find which type of sports drink suits you best.

HOME-MADE SPORTS DRINKS

HYPOTONIC	ISOTONIC
• 20–40 g sucrose 1 litre water 1–1.5 g salt* Flavouring*	• 40–80 g sucrose 1 litre water 1–1.5 g salt* Flavouring*
• 100 ml squash 900 ml water 1–1.5 g salt*	• 200 ml squash 800 ml water 1–1.5 g salt*
• 250 ml fruit juice 750 ml water 1–1.5 g salt*	• 500 ml fruit juice 500 ml water 1–1.5 g salt*

*optional

10
DIETS FOR DIFFERENT SPORTS

The general principles of sports nutrition apply to all sports, but each activity places specific nutritional and energy demands on the body. If you are serious about your sport, you can fine tune your diet to match your individual training programme.

- Each eating plan includes three meals and 2–3 snacks each day. This pattern of eating leads to more efficient glycogen refuelling after exercise and minimises fat deposition.
- In addition to the foods in the menus, you should include a minimum of 2 litres (4 pints) of fluid per day plus ½–1 litre (1–2 pints) for each hour of training. Each pre- and post-workout snack should be accompanied by 150–250 ml water.
- Where one portion of fruit is indicated on the menu, check page 3 for portion sizes.
- All of the menus and recipes serve one person. Simply multiply the amounts by the number of portions if you wish to serve more people.

Long distance running

TIP 1 STAY LEAN
Maintain a low body fat level as excessive weight will reduce your speed and performance. For elite male runners, the optimal body fat range is 5–12%; for elite female runners, the optimal range is 10–18%.

TIP 2 CARB UP
Eating a carbohydrate-rich snack about half an hour before your run can help you exercise longer and more intensively without hitting the wall. Consume 30–60 g/hour during long runs (90+ mins). Try sports drinks, energy bars, energy gels and bananas.

TIP 3 IRON

Keep up your iron intake. Depleted iron stores and iron-deficiency anaemia are particularly common among female runners so include foods detailed on page 61.

LONG DISTANCE RUNNER'S EATING PLAN

Day 1	Breakfast	1 large bowl (75 g/3 oz) wholegrain breakfast cereal 200 ml (⅓ pint) skimmed or semi-skimmed milk 1 banana 1 glass (200 ml/7 fl oz) fruit juice
	Snack	2 slices of Cornmeal Bread (see page 167) or wholemeal bread with honey 1 portion fresh fruit
	Lunch	Brown Rice and Bean Salad (see page 124) 2 wholemeal rolls with butter/low fat spread 2 portions fresh fruit 1 carton (150 g) low fat yoghurt
	Pre-workout snack	75 g (3 oz) raisins or dates
	Post-workout snack	2 Apricot Bars (see page 211)
	Dinner	Potato Tacos (see page 180) 1 thick slice crusty bread Broccoli or other leafy green vegetables 2 portions fresh fruit 1 carton (150 g) low fat fromage frais

Day 2	Breakfast	3 Breakfast Pancakes (see page 192) 1 large glass (250 ml) fruit juice
	Snack	2 cereal or fruit bars
	Lunch	1 large (300 g/11 oz) jacket potato with a little low fat spread 100 g (4 oz) cottage cheese or low fat soft cheese Large mixed salad with 1 tbsp oil/vinegar dressing 1 thick slice bread with butter/low fat spread 2 portions fresh fruit 1 carton (150 g) low fat yoghurt
	Pre-workout snack	400 ml isotonic sports drink (home-made or commercial)
	Post-workout snack	2 Raisin Muffins (see page 225)
	Dinner	Minestrone Soup (see page 115) 2 Corn Muffins (see page 228) 1 tin (400 g) rice pudding 1 tbsp fruit spread or jam
Day 3	Breakfast	4 slices wholemeal toast 1 egg (scrambled/boiled/poached) 2 portions fresh fruit
	Snack	1 cereal or fruit bar (see pages 209–11)
	Lunch	Ciabatta sandwich: 6 slices Ciabatta bread with reduced fat mozzarella, beef tomatoes, olives and low calorie salad dressing 2 portions fresh fruit 1 carton (150 g) low fat fromage frais
	Pre-workout snack	1 energy bar
	Post-workout snack	1 Banana sandwich: 2 slices of bread with 1 sliced banana
	Dinner	Athlete's Hot Pasta with Vegetables (see page 152) Apricot and Date Bread Pudding (see page 220)

Sprinting

TIP 1 GET EXTRA POWER

If you are an experienced or elite sprinter, consider taking creatine supplements. Either a loading dose of 20 g per day (4 x 5 g) for 5 days or a daily 3–6g dose for 30 days can boost muscle phosphocreatine levels. This may help you to maintain your maximal speed longer and recover faster between sets.

TIP 2 MORE PROTEIN

You have higher protein needs compared with endurance runners (1.4–1.8 g/kg per day). Include at least three portions of high protein foods in your daily diet. If you also have very high calorie needs (more than 3000 kcal) you may consider supplementing your diet with a meal-replacement product (see page 42).

SPRINTER'S EATING PLAN

This eating plan provides approximately 3000 kcal per day. Increase or decrease the quantities according to your individual requirements (see above).

Day 1	Breakfast	Power Porridge (see page 194)
	Snack	2 slices Banana Bread (see page 171)
	Lunch	2 Grilled Chicken Burgers (see page 202) 2 portions fresh fruit
	Pre-workout snack	1 piece of fresh fruit 1 fruit bar
	Post-workout snack	Meal replacement shake
	Dinner	Mighty Mash 1 (see page 178) 175 g (6 oz) grilled cod or haddock with herbs Carrots, broccoli or other vegetables 2 portions fresh fruit 1 carton (150 g) low fat fromage frais

Day 2	Breakfast	2 eggs (boiled/scrambled/poached) 4 slices toast with butter/spread I large glass (250 ml) fruit juice
	Snack	Milkshake: 600 ml skimmed/semi-skimmed milk, I banana, 2 tbsp skimmed milk/protein powder
	Lunch	I large (300 g/11 oz) jacket potato 75 g (3 oz) prawns or chicken mixed with I tbsp low calorie salad dressing Large mixed salad with I tbsp dressing 2 portions fresh fruit I carton (150 g) low fat yoghurt
	Pre-workout snack	400 ml isotonic sports drink
	Post-workout snack	3 Oatmeal Cookies (see page 213) I glass (250 ml) skimmed or semi-skimmed milk
	Dinner	Chicken Paella (see page 130) Green beans, courgettes, or other vegetables Baked Bananas (see page 222) I carton (150 g) plain low fat yoghurt
Day 3	Breakfast	4 Weetabix or Shredded Wheat 300 ml (½ pint) skimmed or semi-skimmed milk 25 g (1 oz) dried fruit
	Snack	Bagel Melt (see page 198)
	Lunch	Rice and Sweetcorn Salad (see page 122) 100 g (4 oz) cooked chicken or turkey breast 2 portions fresh fruit I carton (150 g) low fat fromage frais
	Pre-workout Snack	50 g (2 oz) dried fruit
	Post-workout Snack	2 Date and Walnut Bars (see page 210)
	Dinner	75 g (3 oz) pasta (uncooked weight) Vegetarian Bolognese (see page 153) Crunchy Apple Crumble (see page 218) I carton (150 g) low fat yoghurt

Combat sports

TIP 1 STAY CLOSE TO THE MARK

Keep your off-season weight fairly close to your competitive weight. The difference should be no more than about 6 kg (13 lb). If you regularly have difficulty making weight for competition, consider moving up to the next weight category.

TIP 2 MAKE WEIGHT SAFELY

Plan your pre-competition strategy, allowing sufficient time to lose weight safely and slowly (½–1 kg per week). Make weight by losing fat, not fluid and glycogen through starvation or dehydration. Both will have an adverse effect on your performance and health.

COMBAT ATHLETE'S EATING PLAN

This eating plan provides approximately 3000 kcal per day. Increase or decrease the quantities according to your individual requirements (see above).

Day 1	Breakfast	75 g (3 oz) porridge oats 450 ml (¾ pint) skimmed or semi-skimmed milk 1 banana
	Snack	1 wholemeal sandwich: 2 slices bread with a little butter/low fat spread and 50 g (2 oz) lean ham or low fat soft cheese
	Lunch	2 Turkey Pockets (see page 198) 2 portions fresh fruit
	Pre-workout snack	400 ml isotonic sports drink (home-made or commercial)
	Post-workout snack	2 Muesli Bars (see page 209)
	Dinner	Pork and Vegetable Stir Fry (see page 134) 2 portions fresh fruit 1 glass (200 ml) semi-skimmed or skimmed milk

Day 2	Breakfast	1 large bowl (100 g/4 oz) wholegrain breakfast cereal 300 ml (½ pint) skimmed or semi-skimmed milk 1 portion fresh fruit
	Snack	2 large slices toast with fruit spread or honey
	Lunch	Athlete's Cold Pasta Salad (see page 121) 1 thick slice bread with butter/low fat spread 75 g (3 oz) cooked chicken breast or cottage cheese 2 bananas
	Pre-workout snack	50 g (2 oz) dried fruit
	Post-workout snack	1 litre (2 pints) isotonic sports drink
	Dinner	Curried Chicken and Rice (see page 135) 1 tin (400 g) low fat rice pudding 225 g (8 oz) fresh or tinned fruit
Day 3	Breakfast	Raisin Toast (see page 166) 1 large glass (225 ml/8 fl oz) fruit juice
	Snack	2 English muffins with honey
	Lunch	1 large (300 g/11 oz) jacket potato 100 g (4 oz) tinned tuna in brine (drained) mixed with 1 tbsp low fat soft cheese and 1 tbsp reduced fat mayonnaise Tomatoes 1 portion fresh fruit 1 carton (150 g) low fat yoghurt
	Pre-workout snack	2 bananas
	Post-workout snack	1 meal replacement bar
	Dinner	100 g (4 oz) pasta Turkey Bolognese (see page 153) Side salad with 1 tbsp French dressing 2 portions fresh fruit

Weight training and body building

TIP 1 PROTEIN IS KEY

Aim to get between 1.4 and 1.8 g per kg body weight daily, and spread the protein evenly over 5 or 6 meals. An 80 kg bodybuilder would therefore need 112–144 g of protein daily – 22–29 g in each of five meals, or 19–24 g in each of six.

TIP 2 EAT MORE!

To build muscle at the optimum rate, you should increase your calories by 15% over your maintenance requirements. In practice, this means consuming an additional 300–500 kcal per day from a mixture of high carbohydrate and high protein foods.

TIP 3 SUPPLEMENTAL BENEFITS

The majority of supplements marketed for bodybuilders are unnecessary and lacking in scientific evidence – there is no proof that 'andro' supplements or pro-hormones work. Creatine, HMB and glutamine (see page 42) may be beneficial for experienced trainers, and protein/carbohydrate drinks may benefit those with very high calorie and nutritional needs.

BODYBUILDER'S EATING PLAN

This eating plan provides approximately 3000 kcal per day. Increase or decrease the quantities according to your individual requirements (see above).

Day 1	Breakfast	4 Weetabix or Shredded Wheat 300 ml (½ pint) skimmed or semi-skimmed milk 1 banana 1 carton (150 g) low fat yoghurt or fromage frais
	Snack	1 large wholemeal roll with a little butter/low fat spread and 50 g (2 oz) cottage cheese or tuna 1 portion fresh fruit
	Lunch	2 wholemeal pitta breads with 100 g (4 oz) cooked chopped turkey or chicken or 2 sliced boiled eggs, tomatoes and cucumber with 1 tbsp low calorie dressing 1 carton (150 g) low fat yoghurt 1 portion fresh fruit
	Pre-workout snack	50 g (2 oz) dried fruit 200 ml fruit juice (diluted with water)
	Post-workout snack	1 glass (200 ml) semi-skimmed or skimmed milk or a meal-replacement supplement 1 portion fresh fruit Meal replacement shake
	Dinner	Tuna and Pasta Bake (see page 159) Broccoli or other green vegetables Tinned pineapple/peaches 200 ml (⅓ pint) low fat custard
Day 2	Breakfast	300 ml (½ pint) natural yoghurt mixed with 225 g (8 oz) chopped fruit (e.g. strawberries, nectarines, melon) 2 slices toast with honey
	Snack	4 oatcakes 25 g (1 oz) sliced cheese ➡

	Lunch	Omelette 2 eggs and 2 egg whites, filled with 75 g chopped lean ham, sliced tomatoes and mushrooms, and fresh or dried herbs; 2 wholemeal rolls with a little butter/low fat spread 2 portions fresh fruit
	Pre-workout snack	400 ml (⅔ pint) isotonic sports drink (home-made or commercial)
	Post-workout snack	3 slices malt loaf
	Dinner	Foil baked chicken (175 g/6 oz) skinless chicken breast baked in foil with herbs and lemon juice 1 large (300 g/11 oz) jacket potato with 1 tbsp plain yoghurt Vegetable Salad (see page 126) Power Milkshake: 300 ml (½ pint) skimmed milk, 2 tbsp skimmed milk powder or commercial protein powder, 1 carton (150 g) low calorie fruit yoghurt and 1 banana, blended
Day 3	Breakfast	1 glass (150 ml/5 fl oz) fruit juice 2 boiled/poached/scrambled eggs 3 slices wholemeal toast and low fat spread
	Snack	2 fruit or low fat cereal bars 1 glass (200 ml) skimmed or semi-skimmed milk
	Lunch	Curried Chicken Baguette (see page 199) 2 portions fresh fruit
	Pre-workout snack	2 Fruit and Nut Bars (see page 211)
	Post-workout snack	6 rice cakes 1 banana
	Dinner	Quick Tacos (see page 197) 1 jacket potato (225 g/8 oz) with a little butter/low fat spread Side salad 2 portions fresh fruit 1 carton (150 g) low fat fromage frais

Long distance cycling

TIP I REFUEL IN THE SADDLE

For rides lasting longer than 90 minutes, consume between 30–60 g carbohydrate per hour. This will help delay fatigue and improve your endurance. This can be provided by 500 ml isotonic drink (6 g carbohydrate/100 ml) or 2 bananas or 1 energy bar or 50 g (2 oz) raisins.

TIP 2 DRINK SMART

Keep well hydrated as fluid loss during long strenuous rides can be over 1 litre per hour. Drink 125–250 ml water or a sports drink immediately before your ride and 125–150 ml every 10–20 minutes.

This eating plan provides approximately 3000 kcal per day. Increase or decrease the quantities according to your individual requirements (see page 49).

LONG DISTANCE CYCLIST'S EATING PLAN

Day I	Breakfast	I large bowl (100 g/4 oz) bran flakes/wheat flakes /fruit & fibre/muesli 300 ml (½ pint) skimmed or semi-skimmed milk I chopped banana 50 g (2 oz) raisins
	Snack	2 portions fresh fruit 2 slices toast with butter/low fat spread
	Lunch	I large jacket potato (300 g/11 oz) topped with half a large tin (210 g) baked beans Mixed Vegetable Salad (see page 126) with I tbsp oil/vinegar dressing I portion fresh fruit I carton (150 g) low fat yoghurt
	Pre-workout snack	600 ml (I pint) isotonic sports drink (home-made or commercial)
	Post-workout snack	I Oaty Fruit Bar (see page 210)
	Dinner	75 g (3 oz) pasta (uncooked weight) Quick Tuna and Sweetcorn Sauce (see page 155) I tbsp grated cheese Fruit Rice Pudding (see page 218)

Day 2	Breakfast	4 thick slices wholemeal toast with a scraping of low fat spread and 4 heaped tsp fruit spread or honey I glass (175 ml/6 fl oz) fruit juice
	Snack	2 Oatmeal Cookies (see page 213)
	Lunch	Rice and Sweetcorn Salad (see page 122) 2 portions fresh fruit
	Pre-workout snack	2 bananas
	Post-workout snack	Sandwich: 2 slices wholemeal bread with Marmite
	Dinner	Quick vegetable and cheese pizza: I ready-made pizza base (approx. 150–175 g/5–6 oz), 3 tbsp pasta sauce, finely sliced onion, red and green peppers, sliced mushrooms, dried herbs, 50 g (2 oz) grated Cheddar cheese or mozzarella. Bake in a hot oven, according to instructions on the packet I tin (225 g/8 oz) pineapple in juice I carton (150 g) low fat yoghurt
Day 3	Breakfast	75 g (3 oz) porridge oats 450 ml (¾ pint) skimmed or semi-skimmed milk 25 g (1 oz) dates or sultanas
	Snack	I toasted bagel I portion fresh fruit
	Lunch	2 sandwiches: 4 slices wholemeal bread with a little butter/low fat spread and 100 g (4 oz) tuna, tomato, watercress and 2 tbsp low fat salad dressing 2 cartons (300 g) low fat yoghurt
	Pre-workout snack	4 rice cakes spread with 4 tsp fruit spread
	Post-workout snack	I Muesli Bar (see page 209) I banana
	Dinner	Vegetable Paella (see page 131) Tomato salad Banana Bread Pudding (see page 219)

Football, rugby, hockey and other team sports

TIP I CARB UP

Increase your carbohydrate intake during the last 24–48 hours before the day of a match. This will ensure adequate glycogen stores, improve your performance, and reduce the chances of injury.

TIP 2 SNACK ATTACK

Make use of the half-time break, wherever possible, to consume plenty of fluid and a high glycaemic index snack such as bananas, energy or fruit bars. Aim to drink at least 250–300 ml water or an isotonic sports drink after each half of the match.

TEAM SPORT EATING PLAN

This eating plan provides approximately 3000 kcal per day. Increase or decrease the quantities according to your individual requirements (see page 49).

Day I	Breakfast	3 Weetabix or Shredded Wheat 200 ml (⅓ pint) skimmed or semi-skimmed milk I chopped banana
	Snack	I portion fresh fruit I wholemeal roll with 50 g (2 oz) chicken, ham or cheese
	Lunch	4 slices toast I tin (420 g) baked beans Side salad with I tbsp reduced fat dressing I portion fresh fruit I carton (150 g) low fat yoghurt
	Pre-workout snack	600 ml (I pint) isotonic sports drink (home-made or commercial)
	Post-workout snack	2 bananas I roll or English muffin
	Dinner	Spicy Rice (see page 131) I boneless chicken or turkey portion (100 g/4 oz) 2 Raisin Muffins (see page 225)

Day 2	Breakfast	Dried Fruit Muesli (see page 191) 300 ml (½ pint) skimmed or semi-skimmed milk 1 glass (175 ml/6 fl oz) fruit juice
	Snack	1 bagel (any variety) 1 portion fresh fruit
	Lunch	75 g (3 oz) pasta (uncooked weight) Tomato and Tuna Sauce (see page 155) 2 thick slices bread with butter/low fat spread 2 portions fresh fruit
	Pre-workout snack	75 g (3 oz) raisins or dates
	Post-workout snack	2 Oaty Fruit Bars (see page 210)
	Dinner	Chilli Con Carne (see page 150) or Mixed Bean Chilli (see page 148) Large mixed salad with 1 tbsp reduced fat dressing 1 carton (150 g) low fat yoghurt 1 banana
Day 3	Breakfast	75 g (3 oz) porridge oats 450 ml (¾ pint) skimmed or semi-skimmed milk Handful of raisins
	Snack	2 slices toast with butter/low fat spread and Marmite 2 portions fresh fruit
	Lunch	One-minute Burrito (see page 147) Tomatoes, cucumber 2 cartons (300 g) low fat yoghurt
	Pre-workout snack	2 cereal bars (low fat)
	Post-workout snack	4 rice cakes 1 banana
	Dinner	Chicken and Mushrooms with Pasta (see page 162) 1 wholemeal roll with butter/low fat spread Crunchy Apple Crumble (see page 218)

Swimming

TIP 1 SHED THE BLUBBER

Forget the myth that swimmers need extra body fat. Unless you are a very long distance swimmer (e.g. cross-Channel), a lower body fat percentage will improve your performance. Women perform best with a body fat percentage below 25% and men below 15%.

TIP 2 AVOID THE VENDING MACHINE

Swimming often enhances the appetite immediately following exercise. Refuel on low fat high carbohydrate foods such as toast, sandwiches, jacket potatoes, bananas or breakfast cereal, rather than the crisps and chocolate bars frequently on offer at swimming venues.

SWIMMER'S EATING PLAN

This eating plan provides approximately 3000 kcal per day. Increase or decrease the quantities according to your individual requirements (see page 49).

Day 1	Breakfast	75 g (3 oz) wheat or bran flakes 200 ml (⅓ pint) skimmed or semi-skimmed milk 25 g (1 oz) raisins
	Snack	2 portions fresh fruit 2 slices toast with butter/low fat spread
	Lunch	1 large jacket potato (300 g/11 oz) topped with half a large tin (210 g) baked beans Mixed vegetable salad (see page 126) with 1 tbsp oil/vinegar dressing 1 portion fresh fruit 1 carton (150 g) low fat yoghurt
	Pre-workout snack	600 ml (1 pint) isotonic sports drink (home-made or commercial)
	Post-workout snack	2 Oaty Fruit Bars (see page 210)
	Dinner	75 g (3 oz) pasta (uncooked weight) Quick Tuna and Sweetcorn Sauce (see page 155) 50 g (2 oz) grated cheese Fruit Rice Pudding (see page 218)

Day 2	Breakfast	4 thick slices wholemeal toast with a scraping of low fat spread and 4 heaped tsp fruit spread or honey I glass (175 ml/6 fl oz) fruit juice
	Snack	2 Oatmeal Cookies (see page 213)
	Lunch	Rice and Sweetcorn Salad (see page 122) 2 portions fresh fruit
	Pre-workout snack	2 bananas 2 glasses water
	Post-workout snack	Sandwich: 2 slices wholemeal bread with Marmite
	Dinner	Quick vegetable and cheese pizza: I ready-made pizza base (approx. 150–175 g/5–6 oz), 3 tbsp pasta sauce, finely sliced onion, red and green peppers, sliced mushrooms, dried herbs, 50 g (2 oz) grated Cheddar cheese or mozzarella. Bake in a hot oven, according to instructions on the packet I tin (225 g/8 oz) pineapple in juice I carton (150 g) low fat yoghurt
Day 3	Breakfast	I large bowl (100 g/4 oz) muesli 300 ml (½ pint) skimmed or semi-skimmed milk I chopped banana 50 g (2 oz) raisins
	Snack	I toasted bagel I portion fresh fruit
	Lunch	2 sandwiches: 4 slices wholemeal bread with a little butter/low fat spread and 100 g (4 oz) tuna, tomato, watercress and 2 tbsp low fat salad dressing 2 cartons (300 g) low fat yoghurt
	Pre-workout snack	4 rice cakes spread with 4 tsp fruit spread 2 glasses water
	Post-workout snack	I Muesli Bar (see page 209) I banana
	Dinner	Mexican Rice (see page 136) I portion fresh fruit

Aerobics

TIP I EAT SMART ON THE RUN

Plan your diet carefully so you eat at regular intervals (every 2–3 hours) and avoid leaving long gaps between meals. Take a supply of low fat snacks with you if you have to eat on the run, e.g. sandwiches, rolls, cereal and fruit bars, oatcakes, fresh fruit, popcorn, breadsticks, low fat yoghurt. If you exercise for longer than 90 minutes, have at least 500 ml of an isotonic drink to maintain blood sugar levels and prevent dehydration.

TIP 2 VITAMIN HELP

If your eating habits tend to be erratic, consider taking a multi-vitamin and mineral supplement to safeguard against deficient intakes.

AEROBICS EATING PLAN

This eating plan provides approximately 2500 kcal per day. Increase or decrease the quantities according to your individual requirements (see page 49).

Day I	Breakfast	I medium bowl (50 g/2 oz) wholegrain breakfast cereal 150 ml (¼ pint) skimmed or semi-skimmed milk I chopped banana
	Snack	2 portions fresh fruit
	Lunch	A–Z Vegetable Soup (see page 115) 2 wholemeal rolls with a little butter/low fat spread 75 g (3 oz) cottage cheese or tuna I portion fresh fruit I carton (150 g) low fat yoghurt
	Pre-workout snack	4 rice cakes with fruit spread
	Post-workout snack	2 Fruit and Nut Bars (see page 211)
	Dinner	75 g (3 oz) pasta (uncooked weight) Tomato and Herb Sauce (see page 156) Fruit Rice Pudding (see page 218)

Day 2	Breakfast	3 thick slices wholemeal toast with a scraping of low fat spread and 2 heaped tsp fruit spread or honey 1 glass (175 ml/6 fl oz) fruit juice
	Snack	1 Oatmeal Muffin (see page 227) 1 portion fresh fruit
	Lunch	Bean Feast (see page 125) 2 thick slices bread with butter/low fat spread 2 portions fresh fruit
	Pre-workout snack	1 banana
	Post-workout snack	Fruit yoghurt
	Dinner	Stir Fried Rice with Vegetables (see page 134) 1 tin (225 g/8 oz) pineapple in juice 1 carton (150 g) low fat yoghurt
Day 3	Breakfast	Granola (see page 193) 200 ml (⅓ pint) skimmed or semi-skimmed milk 1 portion fresh fruit
	Snack	1 slice of Banana Cake (see page 229) 1 portion fresh fruit
	Lunch	2 sandwiches: 4 slices wholemeal bread with a little butter/low fat spread and 100 g (4 oz) tuna, tomato, watercress and 2 tbsp low fat salad dressing 1 carton (150 g) low fat fromage frais
	Pre-workout snack	1 thick slice bread with honey or jam
	Post-workout snack	1 Muesli Bar (see page 209) 1 banana
	Dinner	Chicken Enchiladas or Spicy Bean Enchiladas (see pages 143–4) 1 medium (225 g/8 oz) jacket potato with yoghurt Side salad with 1 tbsp oil/vinegar dressing Hot Winter Fruit Salad or Cool Summer Fruit Salad (see page 219)

11 COMPETITION COUNTDOWN

Your diet during the week before your competition will have a big effect on your performance, and could provide that edge to help you win. Your nutritional preparation will depend on the type of sport you participate in and the duration of the event. The following guide will help you perform at your best.

Pre-competition

THE WEEK BEFORE

You should aim to fully replenish your glycogen stores during the final week and keep well hydrated. Those competing in endurance events lasting longer than 90 minutes may benefit from carbohydrate loading which involves increasing glycogen levels higher than normal (see below). For shorter events, optimal glycogen levels can be achieved by tapering your training and consuming extra carbohydrate 48–72 hours before the event.

CARBOHYDRATE LOADING

Carbohydrate loading is useful for high-intensity endurance events lasting longer than 90 minutes. It is a technique used to increase glycogen above normal levels. The classical regime involves a three-day depletion phase (low carbohydrate diet/intense training) followed by a three-day loading phase (high carbohydrate diet/tapered training). However, this is often associated with side effects such as tiredness and irritability, so a modified regime, omitting the depletion phase, is now recommended. This simply involves tapered training and a high carbohydrate diet and can produce similar results.

TOP LOADING TIPS

- Practise your competition strategy in training.
- Gradually reduce the amount of training to decrease the use of muscle glycogen. Rest on the day prior to competition.
- Eat extra carbohydrate during the three days prior to competition. Aim to eat 7–10 g/kg body weight per day.
- Avoid high fat foods as they may lead to unwanted fat gain.
- If bloating or feeling overfull is a problem, reduce your fibre intake, choosing more refined cereals and simple carbohydrates, e.g. white bread instead of brown, fruit juice instead of fresh fruit, adding more sugar, jam or preserves to your meals.
- Sports drinks, glucose polymer drinks and meal replacement supplements (shakes and bars) can help boost your carbohydrate intake without adding bulk.

THE DAY BEFORE

The day before the event you should rest or do only very light exercise. Eat a substantial supper high in carbohydrate to top up muscle glycogen stores. Stick to plain foods, such as pasta, potatoes and rice and keep the fat content of the meal to a minimum. Avoid alcohol as it is a diuretic and may leave you dehydrated.

THE PRE-COMPETITION MEAL

Eat your pre-competition meal 2–4 hours before you are due to compete. The aims are to:

- top up liver glycogen levels
- maintain blood sugar levels
- stave off hunger
- maintain hydration.

If you are competing in the morning, eat a light breakfast or snack, high in carbohydrate. For afternoon events, eat a more substantial breakfast followed by a light lunch. For evening events, eat a substantial breakfast and lunch followed by a light snack approximately two hours prior to the event. Some athletes benefit from eating a snack containing approximately 25–50 g carbohydrate less than one hour before the event.

PRE-COMPETITION MEAL GUIDELINES

- Stick to familiar and easily digestible foods.
- Foods should be high in carbohydrate, low in fat and moderate in protein.
- Avoid salty or spicy foods; avoid added salt.
- Foods should be low or moderate in fibre.
- Don't overeat – eat a comfortable amount of food.
- Choose a liquid meal or sports drink if you cannot tolerate solid food.
- Drink fluids liberally – 250–500 ml two hours prior to competition.

Suitable pre-competition meals

PRE-COMPETITION BREAKFAST	PRE-COMPETITION LUNCH	PRE-COMPETITION SNACK
One bowl of breakfast cereal (e.g. Cornflakes, Weetabix) Low fat milk Toast with jam or honey Fresh fruit Water	Pasta with tomato sauce Bread or roll Fruit juice Water	Sandwich with low fat filling Fruit or cereal snack bar
OR	OR	OR
Toast, english muffins, pancakes or bagels with honey Fruit juice and water	Jacket potato (large) with low fat filling Salad (no dressing) Fresh fruit Water	Low fat rice pudding Fresh or tinned fruit

> **DON'T FORGET TO DRINK!**
> Make sure you are well hydrated before the event. Your urine
> should be pale in colour and practically odourless. Consume
> 250–500 ml fluid two hours before the event followed by
> 125–250 ml immediately before the event. Choose water or an
> isotonic sports drink.

During competition

Additional carbohydrate (30–60 g per hour) can benefit performance
during high-intensity events lasting more than 90 minutes. You may be
able to carry solid food or drinks with you (e.g. while cycling) or
arrange pick up points. Suitable choices include:

- energy bars
- home-made snack bars
  (see recipes pages 209–13)
- sports drinks
- bananas
- dried fruit
- glucose tablets
- sweets/sugar
  confectionery
- energy gels

BETWEEN EVENTS/HEATS

If you compete in several events or heats during the day (e.g. track and
field events, swimming heats, tennis tournaments, judo, gymnastics),
small light snacks will help top up glycogen and blood sugar levels
during your rest periods. Aim to eat little and often and avoid long
gaps. Take a good supply of snacks and drinks with you, such as:

- sandwiches
- bread, bagels, buns
- fresh fruit
- low fat yoghurt, rice pudding, fromage frais
- home-made muffins (see pages 225–8)
- home-made snack bars and cookies (see pages 209–13)
- home-made cakes (see pages 229–34)
- rice cakes
- energy bars and fruit bars
- low fat crackers and biscuits (e.g. fig rolls)
- diluted squash or fruit juice
- sports drinks (home-made or commercial)
- water
- ready-to-drink meal replacement shakes

Post-competition

To speed your recovery, refuel and rehydrate as soon as possible after your event. A light snack containing 1 g carbohydrate/kg eaten during the two-hour post-exercise period will promote faster muscle glycogen refuelling. Check the carbohydrate counter (see pages 17–18) for suitable food portions. Choose high GI snacks such as bananas, honey sandwiches and energy bars or, alternatively, a sports drink containing 4–8 g carbohydrate/100 ml. Drink at least 500 ml water or sports drink immediately after the event and continue drinking at regular intervals. Your post-event meal should be high in carbohydrate and contain moderate amounts of fat and protein. Avoid rich and spicy foods as these may cause a stomach upset and delay refuelling.

SUITABLE POST-EVENT MEALS

- Thick crust pizza with vegetable topping.
- Jacket potato filled with beans, fish, chicken or cheese.
- Rice dishes such as risotto, rice salad.
- Pasta dishes (avoid creamy sauces).
- Low fat or vegetable lasagne (see pages 161–2).
- Pasta salads (see chapter 13).

PRE-COMPETITION EATING PLAN

- The following six-day menu is based on the carbohydrate needs of an athlete weighing 70 kg. Days 1–3 provide approximately 7 g carbohydrate/kg; days 4–6 provide approximately 8–10 g carbohydrate/kg. Simply decrease or increase slightly the quantities according to your actual body weight.
- In addition to the foods listed, you should also include a minimum of 2 litres (4 pints) of fluid plus 1 litre (2 pints) for each hour of training. Each pre- and post-workout snack should be accompanied with 150–250 ml of water.
- Where one portion of fruit is indicated, check page 3 for portion sizes.

Day 1	Breakfast	1 large bowl (75 g/3 oz) wholegrain breakfast cereal 200 ml (⅓ pint) skimmed or semi-skimmed milk 50 g (2 oz) dried fruit 1 glass (200 ml/7 fl oz) fruit juice
	Snack	2 slices bread with butter/low fat spread and Marmite 1 portion fresh fruit
	Lunch	Potato and Leek Soup (see page 114) 1 wholemeal roll with butter/low fat spread 50 g (2oz) cottage cheese or ham 2 portions fresh fruit 1 carton (150 g/5 oz) low fat yoghurt
	Pre-workout snack	50 g (2 oz) raisins or dates
	Post-workout snack	2 Muesli Bars (see page 209)
	Dinner	300 g (11 oz) jacket potato 100 g (4 oz) fromage frais or cottage cheese Broccoli or other green vegetables 1 portion fresh fruit
	Snack	2 slices toast with butter/low fat spread 1 glass (200 ml/7 fl oz) skimmed or semi-skimmed milk
Day 2	Breakfast	3 Breakfast Pancakes (see page 192) 1 glass (200 ml/7 fl oz) skimmed or semi-skimmed milk
	Snack	1 Date and Walnut Bar (see page 210) 1 banana

	Lunch	2 sandwiches: 4 thick slices of bread with 75 g (3 oz) turkey or chicken and 2 tbsp low calorie coleslaw 2 portions fresh fruit 1 carton (150 g/5 oz) low fat yoghurt
	Pre-workout snack	400 ml (14 fl oz) isotonic sports drink (home-made or commercial)
	Post-workout snack	2 Raisin Muffins (see page 225)
	Dinner	100 g (4 oz) pasta (uncooked weight) Quick Tuna and Sweetcorn Sauce (see page 155) 1 tbsp grated cheese Fruit Rice Pudding (see page 218)
	Snack	2 Fruit and Nut Bars (see page 211)
Day 3	Breakfast	3 slices wholemeal toast with low fat spread 2 eggs (scrambled/boiled/poached) 1 glass (200 ml/7 fl oz) fruit juice
	Snack	1 banana sandwich: 2 slices of bread with 1 sliced banana and a little honey
	Lunch	300 g (11 oz) jacket potato 100 g (4 oz) sweetcorn with peppers 2 spoonfuls plain yoghurt 2 portions fresh fruit 1 carton (150 g/5 oz) low fat fromage frais
	Pre-workout snack	1 energy bar
	Post-workout snack	2 Raisin Muffins (see page 225)
	Dinner	Athlete's Hot Pasta with Vegetables (see page 152) 2 slices bread with butter/low fat spread Hot Winter Fruit Salad or Cool Summer Salad (see page 219)
	Snack	1 medium bowl (50 g/2 oz) breakfast cereal (any variety) 150 ml (¼ pint) skimmed or semi-skimmed milk

Day 4	Breakfast	1 large bowl (100 g/4 oz) breakfast cereal (any variety) 250 ml (½ pint) skimmed or semi-skimmed milk 1 portion of fresh fruit 50 g (2 oz) raisins
	Snack	1 large roll filled with honey 250 ml (½ pint) isotonic sports drink
	Lunch	2 Banana Hot Dogs (see page 198) ½ tin (200 g) low fat rice pudding 2 tbsp fruit spread or jam
	Pre-workout snack	60 g (2 oz) dried fruit 25 g (1 oz) raisins
	Post-workout snack	2 Oaty Fruit Bars (see page 210)
	Dinner	Hawaiian Rice (see page 132) 150 ml (¼ pint) skimmed or semi-skimmed milk
	Snack	4 rice cakes or low fat crackers 2 tbsp fruit spread or jam
Day 5	Breakfast	4 thick slices toast with 8 heaped tsp fruit spread or honey 1 glass (175 ml/6 fl oz) fruit juice 1 banana
	Snack	2 Oatmeal Cookies (see page 213)
	Lunch	Rice and Sweetcorn Salad (see page 122) 2 thick slices bread 2 portions fresh fruit
	Pre-workout snack	2 cereal/fruit bars
	Post-workout snack	Sandwich: 2 slices of bread and 4 tbsp jam or fruit spread 1 glass (200 ml/7 fl oz) fruit juice
	Dinner	Pizza with extra vegetable toppings (2 portions – see page 205) Banana Bread Pudding (see page 219) 1 glass (200 ml/7 fl oz) fruit juice

Day 6	Breakfast	4 Breakfast Muffins (see page 191) or 3 English muffins 4 tbsp fruit spread or honey 2 bananas
	Snack	1 toasted bagel with 1 tbsp fruit spread or honey 1 portion fresh fruit
	Lunch	Athlete's Cold Pasta Salad (see page 121) 2 thick slices bread 1 portion fresh fruit 1 carton (150 g/5 oz) low fat yoghurt
	Dinner	Vegetable Paella (see page 131) 2 slices bread 2 portions tinned fruit (e.g. peaches, pineapple, apricots)
	Snack	1 medium bowl (50 g/2 oz) breakfast cereal 150 ml (¼ pint) skimmed or semi-skimmed milk
Day 7 (competition day)	Breakfast	1 large bowl (75 g/3 oz) breakfast cereal 200 ml (⅓ pint) skimmed milk 1 banana 50 g (2 oz) raisins
	Pre-race snack (optional)	1 banana or 250 ml (½ pint) isotonic sports drink
	Race snacks (if appropriate – see page 104)	Energy bars 250–600 ml (½–1 pint) isotonic sports drinks (quantity depends on duration of event) 25–75 g (1–3 oz) dried fruit
	Post-race snack	3 Fruit Cookies (see page 212) 250–600 ml (½–1 pint) isotonic sports drink

PART II: RECIPES

Notes on the recipes

All the following recipes have been developed in line with the nutritional recommendations for athletes. They are high in carbohydrate, low in fat and provide a good variety of vitamins and minerals. They have been specifically designed to be quick and easy to prepare, making use of basic, nutritious ingredients and simple preparation methods. Menu plans, which include the recipes, are given throughout the previous chapters.

NUTRITIONAL ANALYSIS

The nutritional analysis provides a breakdown of the calorie, protein, fat, carbohydrate and non-starch polysaccharide (fibre) content per serving. The nutrient values are derived from McCance & Widdowson's *Composition of Foods* (HMSO) and, where appropriate, manufacturer's own data. Figures have been rounded to the nearest whole number.

PORTION SIZES

Most of the recipes make four generous-sized servings. Athletes with particularly high calorie and nutritional requirements may increase the quantities accordingly or eat two portions. You may halve or double the quantities if you wish to serve fewer or more people; alternatively, freeze any remaining portions so you will have a ready-made meal on stand-by.

OPTIONAL INGREDIENTS AND VARIATIONS

In many cases you have the choice of sticking to the basic recipe or adding additional ingredients. There are suggestions for substitutions and variations so you are able to adapt any particular recipe to your individual preferences. Experiment as you go along and feel free to add any of your own favourite ingredients.

12 SOUPS

Many people think of soup as a starter, but with the right ingredients it can be transformed into a substantial main meal. Add nutritious ingredients such as potatoes, grains, vegetables and beans and you have a nutritionally complete meal. It is also a superb way to use up any leftovers. For a quick meal bring some stock to the boil or open a tin of ready-made soup, then simply add extra meat or vegetables or whatever ingredients you have handy. Even preparing a soup from fresh ingredients takes less than 10 minutes. There is no need to serve anything else except some fresh, crusty (preferably wholemeal) bread.

SOUP SAVVY

Make a large quantity of soup – enough for several portions – then store the remainder in the fridge (up to 3 days) or freezer (up to 3 months).

1 Fry an onion in a little olive oil. Then add any of the following ingredients.
  • Root vegetable soup: any combination of chopped carrots, swede, turnips, parsnips.
  • Chicken soup: chopped uncooked chicken, sweetcorn, herbs and milk.
  • Minestrone: tinned tomatoes, chopped carrots, frozen peas, baked beans and dried pasta shells.
  • Vegetable soup: any chopped fresh or leftover vegetables or frozen vegetables, e.g. peas, carrots, cauliflower, green beans.
  • Potato soup: sliced potato and paprika.
  • Lentil soup: red lentils and any variety of vegetables.

2 Add liquid and bring to the boil. Choose from the following:
  • 1 tbsp vegetable stock concentrate dissolved in 600 ml (1 pint) water
  • 1 vegetable/chicken/beef stock cube dissolved in 600 ml (1 pint) water
  • A mixture of milk and water
  • 1 tin of ready-made soup (dilute with extra water if necessary)
  • 1 packet of soup made up with water.

3 Cover the saucepan and simmer until the vegetables or meat are cooked.

4 Get ready to serve.
  • For a smooth soup, liquidise the soup in a blender.
  • For a thick soup, blend half the soup in a blender and return to the pan.
  • For a chunky soup, serve straight from the saucepan.

POTATO AND LEEK SOUP

A great way of getting your vitamins

Makes 4 servings

3 medium potatoes, scrubbed and chopped into chunks
3 large leeks, chopped
1 large carrot, chopped
1 vegetable stock cube or 2 teaspoons Swiss Vegetable Bouillon
450 ml (¾ pint) water
600 ml (1 pint) skimmed milk
Handful of chopped fresh herbs, e.g. parsley, basil, thyme (optional)

1 Place all of the ingredients except the milk in a large saucepan. Bring to the boil and simmer for approximately 20 minutes, or until the vegetables are soft.

2 Remove from the heat, add the milk and liquidise (use a blender, food processor or a hand blender).

3 Return to the saucepan, add some freshly ground black pepper and any fresh herbs. Heat through until just hot.

Per serving		% energy
Energy	152 kcal	
Protein	8.4 g	22%
Fat	0.7 g	4%
Carbohydrate	30 g	74%
Fibre	3.1 g	

'CREAM' OF TOMATO SOUP

Although no cream is used in this recipe, a thick, creamy consistency is achieved by using potato and skimmed milk.

Passata is an excellent source of lycopene, a powerful anti-cancer compound

Makes 4 servings

1 tbsp butter or oil
1 onion, chopped
1 large potato, chopped
2 garlic cloves, crushed
¼ tsp each of dried basil, thyme and dill
Salt and freshly ground black pepper
600 ml (1 pint) passata (smooth sieved tomatoes)
1 tsp sugar
350 ml (12 fl oz) skimmed milk

1 Heat the butter or oil in a large saucepan. Cook the onion, potato, garlic and herbs for 5 minutes.

2 Add the seasoning, passata and sugar. Bring to the boil and simmer for approximately 20 minutes, or until the potatoes are soft. Liquidise the soup.

3 Add the milk and heat through until just hot.

Per serving		% energy
Energy	110 kcal	
Protein	5.3 g	20%
Fat	2.4 g	20%
Carbohydrate	18 g	60%
Fibre	1.8 g	

A–Z VEGETABLE SOUP

A great way of meeting your 5-a-day target for fruit and vegetables

Makes 4 servings

1 onion, chopped
1 garlic clove, crushed
1 l (1¾ pints) vegetable stock or
3½ tsp Swiss Vegetable Bouillon/2
vegetable stock cubes dissolved
in 1 l water
750 g (1½ lb) vegetables of your
choice (see below)
Freshly ground black pepper
1 tsp dried mixed herbs

1 Place the onion, garlic and a little
stock in a large saucepan and cook
for 5 minutes.
2 Add the remaining stock, vegetables,
seasoning and herbs. Bring to the
boil and simmer for approximately
20 minutes, or until the vegetables
are soft.
3 Decide on your preferred
consistency of soup (see page 113)
and liquidise accordingly.

A–Z Vegetables: chopped potato,
sliced courgettes, sliced carrots,
diced pumpkin, chopped green
beans, frozen peas, broccoli florets,
cauliflower florets.

Per serving		% energy
Energy	71 kcal	
Protein	3.5 g	20%
Fat	0.8 g	10%
Carbohydrate	13 g	70%
Fibre	3.6 g	

MINESTRONE SOUP

Haricot beans are packed with protein, iron and zinc

Makes 4 servings

1 onion, chopped
2 garlic cloves, crushed
1 l (1¾ pints) vegetable stock or 3
½ tsp Swiss Vegetable Bouillon/2
vegetable stock cubes dissolved in
1 l water
2 carrots, chopped
225 g (8 oz) other vegetables of
choice, e.g. courgettes, peas, green
beans
2 tsp dried basil
1 tin (400 g) haricot beans
100 g (4 oz) small pasta shapes
600 ml (1 pint) passata (smooth
sieved tomatoes) or tinned
chopped tomatoes

1 Bring the onions and garlic to the
boil in a little of the vegetable stock
and simmer for 5 minutes.
2 Add the vegetables, herbs and
remaining stock and continue to
simmer for 10 minutes.
3 Add the beans, pasta and passata
and continue to cook for a further
10 minutes. Serve hot.

Per serving		% energy
Energy	225 kcal	
Protein	12 g	21%
Fat	1.5 g	6%
Carbohydrate	44 g	73%
Fibre	9.2 g	

SOUPS

BROCCOLI AND BEAN SOUP

This sounds like an unusual combination, but it works really well. The mild-flavoured flageolet beans and potato give the soup a creamy texture, while broccoli is one of the most nutritious vegetables, full of vitamin C, iron, folic acid and cancer-fighting phytochemicals.

Makes 4 servings

4 spring onions, sliced
1 garlic clove, crushed
2 tsp mild curry powder
1 l (1¾ pints) vegetable stock or
3½ tsp Swiss Vegetable Bouillon/2
vegetable stock cubes dissolved
in 1 l water
1 medium potato, chopped
450 g (1 lb) broccoli florets
1 tin (420 g) flageolet beans,
drained

1 Place the onions, garlic and curry powder in a saucepan with 150 ml of the stock. Bring to the boil and simmer for about 5 minutes.

2 Add the remaining stock, the potato and broccoli and simmer for 15–20 minutes.

3 Add the beans, then purée the soup (in small batches if necessary).

Per serving		% energy
Energy	228 kcal	
Protein	12 g	20%
Fat	1.4 g	6%
Carbohydrate	45 g	74%
Fibre	8 g	

PEA AND POTATO SOUP

This simple soup makes a nutritionally complete meal – it is rich in protein, fibre, vitamin C and complex carbohydrate.

Makes 4 servings

1 onion, chopped
2 large potatoes, cubed
1 tbsp oil
1 l (1¾ pts) vegetable stock or 3½ tsp Swiss Vegetable Bouillon/2 vegetable stock cubes dissolved in 1 l water
450 g (1 lb) frozen peas
Handful of fresh herbs, e.g. mint and parsley
Freshly ground black pepper

1 Sauté the onion and potato in the oil for 5 minutes.

2 Add the stock and bring to the boil. Simmer for 5 minutes.

3 Add the peas and continue cooking for a further 5 minutes.

4 Stir in the fresh herbs and season with pepper to taste.

Per serving		% energy
Energy	141 kcal	
Protein	10 g	29%
Fat	1.7 g	11%
Carbohydrate	235 g	60%
Fibre	9.2 g	

LENTIL AND VEGETABLE SOUP

Red lentils are rich in protein, iron and fibre

Makes 4 servings

225 g (8 oz) red lentils
1½ l (3 pints) vegetable stock or
5 tsp Swiss Vegetable Bouillon
dissolved in 1 l water
2 carrots, sliced
1 onion, chopped
2 potatoes, diced
Salt and freshly ground black
pepper
225 g (8 oz) swede/turnips/
parsnips/courgettes/cauliflower/
celery/leek, chopped (optional)

1 Place the lentils in a large saucepan
   with the vegetable stock and boil for
   10 minutes. Alternatively, cook in a
   pressure cooker for 3 minutes then
   release the steam.
2 Add the vegetables if using, bring
   back to the boil and simmer for a
   further 15–20 minutes until the
   vegetables and lentils are soft (or
   cook in the pressure cooker for a
   further 3 minutes).
3 Season with salt and pepper.

Per serving		% energy
Energy	195 kcal	
Protein	14 g	28%
Fat	0.9 g	4%
Carbohydrate	35 g	68%
Fibre	3.7 g	

CORN CHOWDER

Rich in complex carbohydrates and protein

Makes 4 servings

1 onion, chopped
2 tsp olive oil
2 potatoes, diced
600 ml (1 pint) water or vegetable
stock or 2 tsp Swiss Vegetable
Bouillon/1 vegetable stock cube
dissolved in 1 l water
600 ml (1 pint) skimmed milk
1 large tin (420 g) cream-style
corn
Salt and freshly ground black
pepper

1 Sauté the onion in the oil for 5
   minutes.
2 Add the potatoes and the water or
   stock. Bring to the boil and cook for
   10 minutes.
3 Add the remaining ingredients and
   simmer for a further 10 minutes,
   stirring occasionally. Season with
   salt and pepper to taste.

Per serving		% energy
Energy	257 kcal	
Protein	9.8 g	15%
Fat	3.6 g	13%
Carbohydrate	50 g	72%
Fibre	2.7 g	

SOUPS

PASTA AND BEAN SOUP

This hearty, high carbohydrate soup is also rich in protein, vitamins and potassium, and is very low in fat.

Makes 4 servings

1 large onion, chopped
2 celery stalks, chopped
1 tsp paprika
1 tin (400 g) chopped tomatoes
1 l (1¾ pints) vegetable stock
100 g (4 oz) pasta shapes
1 tin (420 g) cannelini or haricot beans, drained
1–2 chopped carrots/100 g (4 oz) chopped cabbage (optional)
Salt and freshly ground black pepper

1 Place the onion, celery, paprika, tomatoes and stock in a large saucepan. Bring to the boil and simmer for 10 minutes until the vegetables are soft.

2 Add the pasta and beans and cook for a further 7–10 minutes. Add any additional vegetables at this stage.

3 Season to taste with salt and pepper.

Per serving		% energy
Energy	218 kcal	
Protein	11 g	20%
Fat	1.2 g	5%
Carbohydrate	44 g	75%
Fibre	7.5 g	

CAULIFLOWER CHEESE SOUP

You can substitute broccoli for the cauliflower if you wish.

 Low in fat yet full of flavour

Makes 4 servings

1 onion, chopped
1 cauliflower, cut into florets
600 ml (1 pint) vegetable stock or 2 tsp Swiss Vegetable Bouillon/1 vegetable stock cube dissolved in 1 l water
600 ml (1 pint) skimmed milk
Salt and freshly ground black pepper
50 g (2 oz) mature Cheddar cheese, grated
2 tbsp grated parmesan (optional)

1 Place the onion, cauliflower and vegetable stock in a saucepan. Bring to the boil and simmer for about 15 minutes until the vegetables are soft.

2 Purée the soup in a blender or food processor until smooth.

3 Return to the saucepan with the milk. Season to taste and heat until just boiling.

4 Stir in the cheese until it melts.

5 Sprinkle with parmesan to serve (if applicable).

Per serving		% energy
Energy	151 kcal	
Protein	13 g	33%
Fat	6.2 g	37%
Carbohydrate	12 g	30%
Fibre	2 g	

SOUPS

BAKED BEAN AND VEGETABLE SOUP

Makes 4 servings

A superb way of using up winter vegetables

1 tbsp olive oil
1 onion, chopped
1 celery stick, chopped
2 carrots, sliced
1 clove garlic, crushed
1 turnip or wedge of butternut squash, chopped
1 tin (420 g) baked beans
75 g (3 oz) frozen green beans or peas
600 ml (1 pint) vegetable stock or 2 tsp Swiss Vegetable Bouillon/1 vegetable stock cube dissolved in 1 l water
2 tbsp parsley, chopped

1 Heat the oil in a large saucepan, add the onion and fry until softened.
2 Add the celery, carrots, garlic and turnip. Cover and cook for 5 minutes.
3 Add the baked beans, green beans and stock. Cover and simmer for 10 minutes until the vegetables are tender.
4 Stir in the parsley.

Per serving		% energy
Energy	142 kcal	
Protein	6.1 g	17%
Fat	3.7 g	23%
Carbohydrate	23 g	60%
Fibre	6.9 g	

CHICKEN AND MUSHROOM SOUP

Makes 4 servings

Rich in carbohydrates and proteins

1 l (1¾ pints) chicken stock or 2 chicken stock cubes dissolved in 1 l water
175 g (6 oz) lean cooked chicken, skinned and chopped
100 g (4 oz) mushrooms, sliced
100 g (4 oz) small pasta shapes
½ tsp dried mixed herbs
Freshly ground black pepper

1 Put the stock in a large saucepan. Bring to the boil.
2 Add the mushrooms, chicken and pasta. Stir well and add the herbs. Cover the pan and simmer for about 5 minutes.
3 Season with the black pepper and serve with baps or rolls.

Per serving		% energy
Energy	184 kcal	
Protein	17 g	38%
Fat	2.9 g	14%
Carbohydrate	24 g	48%
Fibre	1.3 g	

13
SALADS AND DRESSINGS

Traditional salads are unappealing when you've got a hearty appetite and high carbohydrate needs to fulfil. These mega salads, however, have been made into substantial main meals by teaming up the vegetables with high carbohydrate foods such as pasta, rice, grains or pulses.

- Prepare a larger quantity of salad than necessary and keep the remainder in the fridge for up to three days.
- Take individual portions in a plastic box for a portable meal on the go.
- Combine with one of the dressings on pages 127–8 just before serving.

ATHLETE'S COLD PASTA SALAD

This basic recipe can be infinitely varied according to the vegetables you have available. Cold, leftover, cooked vegetables, e.g. carrots, broccoli and peas, are also suitable.

Nutritionally balanced and ideal for refuelling after exercise

Makes 4 servings

350 g (12 oz) pasta shapes
4 large tomatoes, chopped
Vegetables of your choice, e.g. spring onions, peppers, broccoli, celery, radishes
One of the following: 225 g (8 oz) chopped cooked turkey or chicken; 225 g (8 oz) tinned tuna or flaked cooked white fish; 400 g (14 oz) tin red kidney beans
4 tbsp dressing (see pages 127–8)

1 Cook the pasta according to the directions on the packet. Drain and rinse with cold water.

2 Combine the pasta with tomatoes, vegetables and your choice of protein food.

3 Combine with the dressing, if applicable.

Per serving		% energy
Energy	411 kcal	
Protein	27 g	26%
Fat	3.6 g	8%
Carbohydrate	73 g	66%
Fibre	7.1 g	

RICE AND SWEETCORN SALAD

Add dried fruit and chopped toasted nuts for extra vitamins and essential fats

Makes 4 servings

350 g (12 oz) rice
4 spring onions, chopped
2 red peppers, chopped
100 g (4 oz) sultanas
50 g (2 oz) toasted flaked almonds
225 g (8 oz) sweetcorn

1 Cook the rice according to the directions on the packet. Drain if necessary, rinse in cold water, and drain again.
2 Place in a large bowl and combine with the remaining ingredients.

Per serving		% energy
Energy	612 kcal	
Protein	13 g	9%
Fat	13 g	19%
Carbohydrate	119 g	72%
Fibre	4.4 g	

QUICK SUPPER SALAD

Rich in protein and ready in under 3 minutes!

Makes 4 servings

1 tin (420 g) pinto beans (or any other variety)
100 g (4 oz) beansprouts
2 beef tomatoes, chopped
2 sticks celery, sliced
2 tbsp chopped fresh parsley
400 g (14 oz) tinned tuna or 2 tbsp sunflower seeds (optional)

1 Drain and rinse the beans. Combine with the vegetables and parsley.
2 Scatter the tuna or sunflower seeds over the top. Serve with crusty bread.

Per serving		% energy
Energy	99 kcal	
Protein	6.8 g	27%
Fat	0.9 g	8%
Carbohydrate	17 g	65%
Fibre	6.2 g	

NEW POTATO SALAD

New potatoes are great source of vitamin C

Makes 4 servings

900 g (2 lb) new potatoes, washed
4 spring onions, chopped
Handful of fresh herbs: mint, dill, parsley
2 tbsp natural yoghurt
2 tbsp salad cream or reduced fat mayonnaise
225 g (8 oz) baby spinach leaves/100 g (4 oz) chopped cooked ham/4 chopped hard boiled eggs (all optional)

1 Cook the potatoes in boiling water until tender. Drain, and halve any large potatoes.

2 Combine the onions, herbs, yoghurt and salad cream or mayonnaise in a large bowl.

3 Mix with the potatoes. Add any optional ingredients.

Per serving		% energy
Energy	199 kcal	
Protein	4.4 g	9%
Fat	2.6 g	12%
Carbohydrate	42 g	79%
Fibre	2.6 g	

SPICY BULGAR WHEAT SALAD

You could use cous cous instead of the bulgar wheat.

Rich in complex carbohydrates, fibre, B vitamins and iron

Makes 4 servings

225 g (8 oz) bulgar wheat
1.2 l (2 pints) boiling water
1 tbsp olive oil
2 tbsp lemon juice
4 spring onions, chopped
2 tsp curry powder
4 tomatoes, chopped
1 tsp each of fresh chopped mint and parsley
Salt and freshly ground black pepper
50 g (2 oz) raisins/50 g (2 oz) cashew nuts/4 chopped hard boiled eggs/100 g (4 oz) chopped cooked chicken (all optional)

1 Place the bulgar wheat in a large bowl and pour on the boiling water. Leave for 30 minutes, then drain.

2 Mix together the olive oil, lemon juice and curry powder. Combine with the bulgar wheat.

3 Add the remaining ingredients and mix together.

Per serving		% energy
Energy	246 kcal	
Protein	6.4 g	10%
Fat	4.2 g	15%
Carbohydrate	47 g	75%
Fibre	1.5 g	

SALADS AND DRESSINGS

123

BROWN RICE AND BEAN SALAD

Brown rice contains four times more fibre than white rice, as well as B vitamins and iron, which are lacking in white rice.

Makes 4 servings

175 g (6 oz) brown rice
1 tin (420 g) red kidney beans
1 red pepper, chopped
2 celery sticks, chopped
4 spring onions, chopped
3 tbsp parsley, chopped
Salt and freshly ground black pepper
Dash of soy sauce
50 g (2 oz) cashew nuts or walnuts/100 g (4 oz) flaked tinned tuna/chopped tomatoes/cooked peas (all optional)

1 Cook the rice in boiling water for 30–40 minutes until tender. Drain and rinse in cold water.

2 Put the rice in a bowl and combine with the remaining ingredients.

Per serving		% energy
Energy	249 kcal	
Protein	8.9 g	14%
Fat	2 g	7%
Carbohydrate	52 g	79%
Fibre	6.7 g	

THREE GRAIN SALAD

Full of slow-release carbohydrates – perfect for carbohydrate loading

Makes 4 servings

100 g (4 oz) brown rice
100 g (4 oz) pearl barley
50 g (2 oz) cous cous
225 g (8 oz) sweetcorn
4 tomatoes, chopped
Red or green pepper/spring onions/courgettes/carrot (all optional)

1 Cover the rice in plenty of boiling water and cook for 10 minutes. Add the barley and continue to cook for a further 20 minutes. Finally, add the cous cous and cook for another 5 minutes. Add more water if necessary. Drain and rinse briefly in cold water.

2 Mix the grains together in a bowl and combine with the sweetcorn, tomatoes and any optional ingredients.

Per serving		% energy
Energy	375 kcal	
Protein	8.5 g	9%
Fat	2.6 g	6%
Carbohydrate	85 g	85%
Fibre	2.2 g	

BEAN FEAST

Rich in protein, B vitamins and iron

Makes 4 servings

225 g (8 oz) green beans, cut
into 5 cm (2 in) lengths
2 tins (2 x 420 g) mixed beans
I tbsp olive oil
2 tbsp white wine vinegar
100 g (4 oz) baby spinach leaves

I Boil or steam the green beans for
approximately 4 minutes or until
just tender. Refresh in cold water
and drain.

2 Mix together the green beans,
drained tinned beans, olive oil and
vinegar.

3 Place the spinach leaves in the
bottom of the serving bowl and pile
the bean mixture on top.

Per serving		% energy
Energy	200 kcal	
Protein	12 g	25%
Fat	5.3 g	24%
Carbohydrate	28 g	51%
Fibre	10 g	

BEAN AND TUNA SALAD

Less than 10 minutes to prepare!

Makes 4 servings

2 tins (2 × 420 g) cannelini or
butter beans, drained
2 celery sticks, chopped
200 g (7 oz) tinned tuna
100 g (4 oz) green beans, cooked
2 tbsp red wine vinegar
I tbsp olive oil
Handful of fresh herbs: chives,
parsley

I Combine the beans, celery, tuna and
green beans in a bowl.

2 Mix together the vinegar, oil and
herbs and combine with the salad.

Per serving		% energy
Energy	195 kcal	
Protein	20 g	40%
Fat	4.2 g	20%
Carbohydrate	21 g	40%
Fibre	7.8 g	

SALADS AND DRESSINGS

ORIENTAL CHICKEN NOODLE SALAD

You can substitute prawns or tofu for the chicken.

Makes 4 servings

3 tbsp soy sauce
2 garlic cloves, crushed
1 tbsp oil (preferably sesame)
300 g (11 oz) chicken fillet, cut into strips
350 g (12 oz) noodles
400 g (14 oz) mange tout
225 g (8 oz) beansprouts
200 g (7 oz) Chinese leaves, chopped
225 g (8 oz) carrots, grated
Lemon juice

1 Combine the soy sauce, garlic cloves and oil in a bowl. Add the chicken, stir to coat, and leave to marinate in the fridge for 1 hour or longer.
2 Cook the noodles according to the directions on the packet. Drain.
3 In a large bowl, combine the noodles, mange tout, beansprouts, carrots and Chinese leaves.
4 Dry fry the chicken in a non-stick pan until cooked through. Toss in the salad and season with the lemon juice.

Per serving		% energy
Energy	539 kcal	
Protein	32 g	24%
Fat	12 g	20%
Carbohydrate	81 g	56%
Fibre	6.7 g	

TWENTY QUICK AND EASY VEGETABLE SALADS

Vegetable salads are simple to make, often need no cooking and are bursting with vitamins, minerals and antioxidant nutrients. Adjust the quantities of the ingredients according to what you have available and to your own preferences. Toss in one of the dressings listed above and serve with some bread or baked potatoes.

1 Baby spinach, watercress, fresh herbs and radicchio.
2 Lambs lettuce, rocket and endive.
3 Cucumber, tomatoes, olives, spring onions, cubed feta cheese.
4 Lightly cooked broccoli florets, mange tout, mixed lettuce leaves, flaked tuna and strips of red and yellow peppers.
5 Grated carrot, cucumber, raisins and walnuts.
6 Bean sprouts, red pepper, celery, parsley, spring onions, chives.
7 Mixed salad leaves, avocado, steamed green beans, chopped walnuts.
8 Shredded cabbage, desiccated coconut, chopped pineapple and grapes.
9 Chicory, orange segments and dates.
10 Cooked pasta, tomato, peppers, red kidney beans.
11 Cooked rice, sweetcorn, cucumber, mushrooms and flaked tuna.
12 Mixed tinned beans (e.g. red kidney beans, borlotti, chick peas), celery and fresh herbs.
13 Tomatoes, spring onions, cucumber, fresh mint and parsley.
14 Fennel, watercress, orange segments and fresh parsley.
15 Avocado, orange segments, chicory, pine nuts.
16 Curly endive, watercress, avocado and sesame seeds.
17 Courgettes, celery, green pepper, spring onions and grapes.
18 Beansprouts, grated carrot, shredded coconut, dates.
19 Cauliflower, watercress, sesame seeds.
20 Sautéed aubergine slices, plain yoghurt, garlic, fresh parsley.

SALADS AND DRESSINGS

DRESS UP A SALAD

A tasty dressing transforms a salad or plate of vegetables and is a great way of getting essential oils. Here are some ideas for quick dressings:

- a drizzle of balsamic vinegar or flavoured vinegar, e.g. raspberry, rosemary, basil, garlic
- a squeeze of lime or lemon juice
- low fat fromage frais mixed with a little mint sauce
- plain yoghurt mixed with lemon juice
- fromage frais with a little wholegrain mustard
- equal quantities of pesto and yoghurt
- low fat salad dressing or mayonnaise mixed with curry powder

GARLIC AND HERB DRESSING

You can add any fresh herbs – such as oregano, basil or marjoram.

50 ml (2 fl oz) red wine vinegar
2 tbsp orange juice
1 tbsp extra virgin olive oil
1 crushed garlic clove
1 tbsp chopped fresh parsley
1 tbsp chopped fresh tarragon

- Place the ingredients in a screw-top jar and shake well to combine.

Serving suggestions: as a dressing for lettuce and other green salads; on coleslaw, with avocado; with steamed green vegetables such as broccoli and green beans.

Per serving (¼ recipe)		% energy
Energy	30 kcal	
Protein	0.2 g	3%
Fat	2.8 g	85%
Carbohydrate	0.8 g	12%
Fibre	0.1 g	

ITALIAN DRESSING

50 ml (2 fl oz) balsamic vinegar
2 tbsp water
2 tsp olive oil
2 tsp capers
1 tbsp chopped fresh oregano or 1 tsp dried oregano
Pinch of salt

- Place the ingredients in a screw-top jar and shake well to combine.

Serving suggestions: as a dressing for potato salad or coleslaw; as a dip for raw vegetable crudités.

Per serving (¼ recipe)		% energy
Energy	22 kcal	
Protein	0.2 g	3%
Fat	2.1 g	86%
Carbohydrate	0.7 g	11%
Fibre	0 g	

SALADS AND DRESSINGS

SALADS AND DRESSINGS

TANGY YOGHURT DRESSING

2 fl oz plain yoghurt
2 tbsp orange juice
1 tbsp honey
2 tsp Dijon mustard
¼ tsp ground ginger

- Thoroughly combine all the ingredients together in a bowl.

Serving suggestions: as a dressing for potato salad, coleslaw or pasta salad; as a dip for raw vegetable crudités.

Per serving (¼ recipe)		% energy
Energy	22 kcal	
Protein	0.8 g	15%
Fat	0.1 g	5%
Carbohydrate	4.7 g	80%
Fibre	0 g	

CUCUMBER AND LIME DRESSING

200 g (7 fl oz) low fat plain yoghurt
1 tsp white wine vinegar
1 tsp lime juice
1 tsp lime zest
1 small cucumber, seeded and finely chopped

- Thoroughly combine all the ingredients together in a bowl.

Serving suggestions: as a dressing for potato salad, coleslaw or pasta salad; as a dip for raw vegetable crudités.

Per serving (¼ recipe)		% energy
Energy	31 kcal	
Protein	2.8 g	36%
Fat	0.4 g	13%
Carbohydrate	4.2 g	51%
Fibre	0.2 g	

SPICY DRESSING

2 tbsp reduced fat mayonnaise
2 tbsp plain low fat yoghurt
Few drops of chilli sauce (to taste)
Chopped fresh coriander (optional)

- Thoroughly combine all the ingredients together in a bowl.

Serving suggestions: as a dressing for chunky vegetable salads; to accompany your favourite sandwich fillings.

Per serving (¼ recipe)		% energy
Energy	52 kcal	
Protein	0.9 g	7%
Fat	4.3 g	76%
Carbohydrate	2.4 g	17%
Fibre	0 g	

14

RICE AND OTHER GRAINS

Rice is a staple of Asian, Far Eastern and Mediterranean diets, which are among the healthiest in the world. It is high in complex carbohydrates, making it the ideal fuel for athletes. Brown rice contains small amounts of B vitamins and fibre but white rice contains very little. The following recipes should inspire you to make rice a regular part of your diet.

TEN WAYS TO MAKE RICE MORE INTERESTING

1 Add a handful of raisins or currants to cooked rice.
2 Cook the rice in chicken or vegetable stock instead of water.
3 Stir a handful of chopped fresh herbs (e.g. parsley, basil, dill, oregano) into cooked rice.
4 Add the grated rind and juice of a lime, lemon or orange to cooked rice.
5 Cook the rice with a tablespoon of curry powder or turmeric.
6 Add some frozen mixed vegetables or peas during the last five minutes of cooking.
7 Add some soy sauce to cooked rice.
8 Cook the rice with a little paprika and chilli powder.
9 Stir a little French dressing (low fat if you prefer) into cold cooked rice.
10 Add a handful of toasted chopped nuts (e.g. almonds, peanuts) or seeds (e.g. sunflower, pumpkin) to cooked rice.

COOKING RICE

Allow about 75 g (3 oz)/half a cup of rice per average portion. There are two basic ways to cook rice:

1. The absorption method

A measured quantity of rice is cooked with a measured quantity of cold water in a covered saucepan until all of the liquid has been absorbed. Do not stir until the end of the cooking time, then fluff up the rice with a fork. The quantity of water and cooking time depends on the variety of rice.

Easy cook rice: 1 part rice to 2 parts water. Cooking time 18–20 minutes.

Basmati rice: 1 part rice to 1½ parts water. Cooking time 12 minutes.

Brown rice: 1 part rice to 2 parts water. Cooking time 35–45 minutes.

Risotto or arborio rice: 1 part rice to 3 parts water. Cooking time 20–25 minutes.

2. The boiling method

Add enough boiling water to the rice to cover it by at least 2½ cm (1 in). Cover and simmer until tender, adding extra water if necessary to keep the rice very moist. At the end of cooking drain the surplus water.

CHICKEN PAELLA

Low in fat and high in protein and carbohydrates

Makes 4 servings

2 chicken breast fillets, skinned and cut into strips
1 tsp olive oil
350 g (12 oz) white rice
Pinch of turmeric
1½ l (2½ pints) chicken stock
8 large uncooked prawns
175 g (6 oz) frozen peas
Salt and freshly ground black pepper

1 Heat the oil in a heavy-based saucepan. Stir fry the chicken for 1 minute over a high heat, just enough to crisp the outside.

2 Add the rice, turmeric and stock, bring to the boil, reduce the heat and simmer for 12 minutes until most of the liquid has been absorbed.

3 Add the prawns and peas and continue to cook for a further 3–5 minutes. Season with salt and pepper.

Per serving		% energy
Energy	460 kcal	
Protein	25 g	22%
Fat	6.8 g	13%
Carbohydrate	79 g	65%
Fibre	2.6 g	

VEGETABLE PAELLA

This is a vegetarian version of the classic Spanish paella which uses vegetables instead of fish. The peas add protein to the dish.

Makes 4 servings

2 tbsp olive oil
1 onion, chopped
2 garlic cloves, crushed
4 celery sticks, chopped
1 red, yellow and green pepper, sliced
1 tsp paprika
350 g (12 oz) rice
1 tin (400 g) chopped tomatoes
900 ml (1½ pints) vegetable stock (or water plus 2 vegetable stock cubes)
225 g (8 oz) frozen peas
Salt and pepper to taste
2 tbsp chopped parsley/50 g (2 oz) black olives (optional)

1 Heat the oil in a large pan and sauté the onion, garlic, celery and peppers for 5 minutes.

2 Add the paprika and rice and stir for another 2–3 minutes.

3 Add the tomatoes and stock, bring to the boil then simmer for 15–20 minutes, until the liquid has been absorbed.

4 Add the peas, season to taste, and heat through for a few more minutes.

5 Stir in the optional ingredients.

Per serving		% energy
Energy	483 kcal	
Protein	12 g	10%
Fat	10 g	19%
Carbohydrate	92 g	71%
Fibre	7 g	

SPICY RICE

To balance the meal serve with pan-fried fish

Makes 4 servings

350 g (12 oz) white rice
2 l (3½ pints) water or stock
2 tsp medium curry powder
225 g (8 oz) mixed frozen vegetables (e.g. peas, carrots, cauliflower)
50 g (2 oz) currants

1 Place the rice, water and curry powder in a large saucepan. Bring to the boil and simmer for 12 minutes, or until the rice is tender and most of the liquid has been absorbed.

2 Add the frozen vegetables and cook for a further 3 minutes.

3 Stir in the currants and heat through before serving.

Per serving		% energy
Energy	399 kcal	
Protein	8.6 g	9%
Fat	3.5 g	8%
Carbohydrate	89 g	83%
Fibre	0.6 g	

RICE AND OTHER GRAINS

CHICKEN AND PEPPER RISOTTO

You can use tinned tuna or cooked turkey instead of the chicken.

Makes 4 servings

2 l (3½ pints) chicken or vegetable stock
350 g (12 oz) white rice
2 peppers, preferably one red, one yellow, cut into thin strips
100 g (4 oz) cooked chicken, chopped
25 g (1 oz) parmesan, grated
Handful of fresh chives or parsley, if available

1 Place the stock, rice and peppers in a large saucepan.
2 Bring to the boil and simmer for 12–15 minutes, until the rice is tender and the liquid has been absorbed.
3 Add the chicken and half the parmesan. Heat through for a few minutes.
4 Serve topped with remaining parmesan and herbs.

Per serving		% energy
Energy	438 kcal	
Protein	19 g	17%
Fat	7 g	14%
Carbohydrate	80 g	69%
Fibre	1.7 g	

HAWAIIAN RICE

To balance the meal serve with grilled chicken or fish

Makes 4 servings

2 l (3½ pints) vegetable stock
350 g (12 oz) white rice
1 onion, chopped
½ tsp turmeric
225 g (8 oz) tin chopped pineapple, drained
50 g (2 oz) currants

1 Place the stock, rice, onion and turmeric in a large saucepan.
2 Bring to the boil, reduce the heat, cover and simmer for 12–15 minutes, until the rice is tender and the liquid has been absorbed.
3 Add the pineapple and currants. Heat through before serving.

Per serving		% energy
Energy	407 kcal	
Protein	7.1 g	7%
Fat	3.2 g	7%
Carbohydrate	93 g	86%
Fibre	1.1 g	

CHINESE FRIED RICE

This healthy adaptation is lower in fat than the classic Chinese version. Add any vegetables or protein foods you have handy to make this a one-dish meal.

Makes 4 servings

350 g (12 oz) rice
1 tbsp olive oil
1 onion, chopped
1 red pepper, chopped
2 eggs
2 tbsp soy sauce
Mushrooms, peas, green beans, peppers, sweetcorn (optional vegetables)
Prawns, chicken, tofu, almonds (optional protein foods)

1 Cook the rice in approximately twice its volume of water.

2 Meanwhile, heat the oil in a wok and fry the onion and pepper for 2–3 minutes. Add any additional vegetables and protein foods and fry for a further 2 minutes (or until the meat is cooked). Push the vegetables to the sides of the wok.

3 Beat the eggs in a dish then pour into the wok and scramble them until just set.

4 Stir in the cooked rice and soya sauce and combine all the ingredients together.

Per serving		% energy
Energy	425 kcal	
Protein	11 g	11%
Fat	9.3 g	20%
Carbohydrate	79 g	69%
Fibre	1.2 g	

THAI CHICKEN AND RICE

You can use any of the available ready prepared stir fry sauces in this recipe.

Makes 4 servings

2 tsp olive oil
4 spring onions (or 1 small onion), chopped
2 boneless breasts of chicken, chopped
100 g (4 oz) mushrooms, sliced
1 small jar (280 g) Thai Stir Fry sauce
2 l (3½ pints) water
350 g (12 oz) white rice
1 red pepper, chopped/50 g (2 oz) water chestnuts, sliced/100 g (4 oz) mange tout/100 g (4 oz) courgettes, sliced (all optional)

1 Heat the oil in a wok.

2 Sauté the onions for 2 minutes then add the chicken and sauté for a further 3 minutes. Then add the mushrooms and any optional vegetables, stirring constantly until they are tender crisp.

3 Stir in the Thai sauce.

4 Meanwhile, cook the rice in the water for approximately 15 minutes, according to instructions on the packet.

5 Combine the cooked rice and Thai chicken.

Per serving		% energy
Energy	484 kcal	
Protein	18 g	15%
Fat	7.1 g	13%
Carbohydrate	93 g	72%
Fibre	0.8 g	

RICE AND OTHER GRAINS

PORK AND VEGETABLE STIR FRY

You can use chicken, turkey or tofu instead of the pork.

Makes 4 servings

1 tsp oil
350 g (12 oz) lean trimmed pork fillet
1 red pepper, sliced
225 g (8 oz) broccoli florets
100 g (4 oz) green beans
1 small jar (280 g) stir fry sauce, e.g. sweet and sour, Thai stir fry, yellow bean
450 g (1 lb) noodles

1 Heat the oil in a wok.
2 Add the pork and stir fry for 4–5 minutes until brown and tender.
3 Add the vegetables to the wok and continue to stir fry for 2–3 minutes. The vegetables should still be crisp.
4 Add the jar of sauce and cook for 1 minute to heat through.
5 Cook the noodles according to the directions on the packet.
6 Spoon the pork and vegetable mixture over the hot noodles.

Per serving		% energy
Energy	593 kcal	
Protein	28 g	19%
Fat	12 g	19%
Carbohydrate	99 g	62%
Fibre	5.9 g	

STIR FRIED RICE WITH VEGETABLES

A great way of adding vegetables to your diet – use seasonal vegetables

Makes 4 servings

1 tbsp olive oil
1 small onion or 4 spring onions, chopped
450 g (1 lb) vegetables: mange tout, broccoli florets, mushrooms, red, green or yellow peppers, water chestnuts, aubergine
50 g (12 oz) rice (uncooked weight), cooked according to directions on the packet
2 tbsp light soy sauce

1 Heat the oil in a wok. Add the onions and other vegetables and stir fry for 4–5 minutes depending on their size.
2 Add the cooked rice and mix together, separating the grains.
3 Add the soy sauce and heat through.

Per serving		% energy
Energy	406 kcal	
Protein	10 g	10%
Fat	6.6 g	15%
Carbohydrate	82 g	75%
Fibre	3 g	

CURRIED CHICKEN AND RICE

Make this dish as substantial as you like by adding extra vegetables. Adjust the amount of curry paste according to your taste!

Makes 4 servings

1 tbsp butter or olive oil
450 g (1 lb) boneless chicken, cut into strips
1 onion, chopped
2 tbsp mild curry paste
350 g (12 oz) rice
600 ml (1 pint) stock or water
1 tin (400 g) tomatoes
350 g (12 oz) vegetables of your choice (e.g. cauliflower, peas, carrots)
50 g (2 oz) sultanas

1 Heat the butter or oil in a large heavy-bottomed pan and cook the chicken strips for 5 minutes until brown. Put aside on a plate.

2 Add the onion and stir-fry for a few minutes.

3 Add the curry paste, rice, stock, tomatoes and vegetables, stir, then bring to the boil. Simmer for 15 minutes.

4 Return the chicken to the pan, add the sultanas and warm through.

Per serving		% energy
Energy	588 kcal	
Protein	36 g	25%
Fat	10 g	15%
Carbohydrate	95 g	60%
Fibre	4.5 g	

BEANS 'N' RICE

This is a vegetarian adaptation of a traditional West Indian dish. The combination of beans and rice increases the overall protein value of the dish.

Makes 4 servings

1 tbsp oil
1 onion, chopped
1 green chilli, seeded and finely chopped
350 g (12 oz) rice
900 ml (1½ pints) vegetable stock (or water plus 2 vegetable stock cubes)
2 large tomatoes, sliced
1 tin (420 g) beans*
50 g (2 oz) creamed coconut
2 tbsp fresh chopped coriander or parsley
* Either red kidney beans, aduki, cannelini, haricot or black beans.

1 Heat the oil in a heavy-bottomed pan and fry the onion for about 5 minutes. Add the chilli and rice and fry for a further 2 minutes.

2 Add the stock and tomato, bring to the boil and simmer for 10 minutes.

3 Add the beans and a little extra water if the mixture looks dry. Cover and cook for a further 5 minutes until the rice is cooked.

4 Stir in the coconut until it is melted and then stir in the coriander or parsley.

Per serving		% energy
Energy	500 kcal	
Protein	13 g	10%
Fat	12 g	21%
Carbohydrate	92 g	69%
Fibre	5.6 g	

RICE AND OTHER GRAINS

135

RICE WITH HADDOCK AND PEAS

Makes 4 servings

350 g (12 oz) stir-fry rice
600 ml (1 pint) vegetable stock
(or 1 tsp Swiss Vegetable
Bouillon/2 vegetable stock cubes
dissolved in 1 l water)
1 bay leaf
350 g (12 oz) haddock fillet
200 g (7 oz) frozen peas
Salt and freshly ground black
pepper

1 Place the rice in a large pan with the stock and bay leaf and bring to the boil. Cover and simmer for 15 minutes.
2 Add the haddock and peas and continue cooking for a further 5 minutes until the liquid has been absorbed and the fish flakes easily. Roughly break up the fish and stir the rice mixture to distribute evenly.
3 Serve with watercress or a green salad.

Per serving		% energy
Energy	441 kcal	
Protein	26 g	24%
Fat	4.1 g	8%
Carbohydrate	80 g	6.8%
Fibre	2.9 g	

MEXICAN RICE

Serve with wholemilk plain yoghurt and chopped fresh coriander

Makes 4 servings

2 tbsp olive oil
1 large onion, chopped
1 green chilli, deseeded and
chopped
2 celery stalks, chopped
2–3 garlic cloves, crushed
2 tsp ground cumin
1 red and 1 green pepper,
chopped
½ tin (200 g) chopped tomatoes
350 g (12 oz) brown rice
600 ml (1 pint) water
1 tin (400 g) sweetcorn, drained
Salt and freshly ground black
pepper
75 g (3 oz) raisins/1 tin (400 g) red
kidney beans (optional)

1 Heat the oil in a large saucepan and sauté the onion, chilli, celery and garlic over a gentle heat until the onion is softened.
2 Stir in the cumin, pepper and tomatoes and cook for a further 2 minutes.
3 Add the rice and water. Bring to the boil, cover and simmer for about 35 minutes until the rice is cooked and liquid absorbed.
4 Stir in the sweetcorn and any optional ingredients, season to taste and heat through.

Per serving		% energy
Energy	522 kcal	
Protein	10 g	8%
Fat	9.7 g	17%
Carbohydrate	105 g	75%
Fibre	5.4 g	

THAI-STYLE GREEN FISH CURRY

To balance the meal serve with a simple green salad or watercress

Makes 4 servings

1 tbsp olive oil
1 onion, thinly sliced
40 g (1½ oz) Thai green curry paste
300 ml (½ pint) coconut milk
450 g (1 lb) firm white fish, e.g. cod or monkfish, cut into chunks
350 g (12 oz) rice
Grated zest of 1 lime

1 Heat the oil in a wok and stir-fry the onion for 3 minutes.

2 Stir in the curry paste, then add the coconut milk. Simmer for about 10 minutes.

3 Add the fish and cook, stirring, for a few minutes.

4 Cook the rice separately, according to the instructions on the packet and serve topped with the fish curry and garnished with the lime zest.

Per serving		% energy
Energy	463 kcal	
Protein	26 g	22%
Fat	6.8 g	13%
Carbohydrate	80 g	65%
Fibre	0.6 g	

QUICK VEGETABLE CURRY

A bit of a cheat's curry, but many of the ready-prepared curry sauces are low in fat and taste almost as good as home-made. Vary the curry with different combinations of vegetables.

Makes 4 servings

1 tbsp oil
1 onion, sliced
1 small jar (300 g) low fat curry sauce, e.g. Dopiaza, Balti, Jalfreizi
700 g (1½ lb) any chopped vegetables, e.g. carrots, turnips, swede, potato, green beans

1 Heat the oil in a large pan. Add the onion and cook over a high heat for 5 minutes.

2 Add the sauce and the prepared vegetables, stirring well.

3 Cover and cook for about 15 minutes until the vegetables are just tender.

4 Serve with cooked rice or ready-bought chappatis and plain thick yoghurt.

Per serving		% energy
Energy	480 kcal	
Protein	8.7 g	7%
Fat	11 g	20%
Carbohydrate	93 g	73%
Fibre	5.4 g	

RICE AND OTHER GRAINS

137

TOFU AND MUSHROOM STIR FRY

Makes 4 servings

Marinade:
   2 tbsp soy sauce
   2 tbsp dry sherry
   1 tbsp vinegar

A nutritionally balanced meal

Stir fry:
   350 g (12 oz) tofu, cubed
   1 tbsp olive oil
   2 garlic cloves, crushed
   2 cm piece fresh ginger, chopped
   1 red pepper, chopped
   4 spring onions, chopped
   225 g (8 oz) mushrooms, sliced
   100 g (4 oz) beansprouts
   1 tsp cornflour
   350 g (12 oz) Chinese noodles

1 Mix the marinade ingredients together, add the tofu, turn a few times and leave for 30 minutes or longer.

2 Heat the oil in a wok and stir fry the garlic and ginger for 1 minute. Add the red pepper, spring onions, mushrooms and beansprouts and stir fry for 2 minutes.

3 Drain the tofu. Blend the marinade with the cornflour, pour over the vegetables and stir quickly until the sauce has thickened. Transfer onto a serving dish.

4 Stir fry the tofu in the wok for 1 minute, turning frequently, and arrange on the vegetables.

5 Cook the noodles according to directions on the packet and serve with the vegetables.

Per serving		% energy
Energy	473 kcal	
Protein	20 g	17%
Fat	12 g	24%
Carbohydrate	72 g	59%
Fibre	4.4 g	

NOODLES WITH SALMON IN FOIL

This complete meal comes in a neat packet; just pop in the ingredients, put it in the oven and let all the flavours blend together.

Makes 1 serving

75 g (3 oz) egg noodles, cooked according to directions on the packet
1 carrot, thinly sliced
2 spring onions, sliced
4 mushrooms
1 salmon steak (about 175 g/6 oz)
Fresh chopped parsley

1 Place the cooked noodles onto the centre of a piece of oiled foil approximately 50 × 30 cm (20 × 12 in).

2 Lay the vegetables and salmon on top. Sprinkle with salt and parsley.

3 Fold the foil over to enclose the salmon and seal the edges. Place on a baking tray.

4 Bake at 180°C/350°F/ gas mark 4 for 15 minutes.

5 Turn onto a plate to serve.

Per serving		% energy
Energy	681 kcal	
Protein	47 g	28%
Fat	27 g	35%
Carbohydrate	68 g	37%
Fibre	4.7 g	

STIR FRY INDONESIAN PRAWNS IN PEANUT SAUCE

For a vegetarian version, replace the prawns with firm tofu, cut into cubes.

Makes 4 servings

225 g (8 oz) green beans, cut in half cross-ways
450 g (1 lb) large peeled prawns
75 g (3 oz) chunky peanut butter
150 ml (¼ pint) unsweetened canned coconut milk
1 tbsp soy sauce
2 tsp curry powder
350 g (12 oz) Chinese noodles, cooked
A few spring onions, chopped (optional)

1 Place a wok over a high heat. Add the green beans and prawns and stir fry for 3 minutes.

2 In a small bowl, whisk together the peanut butter, coconut milk, soy sauce, curry powder and 175 ml (6 fl oz) water.

3 Pour over the beans and prawns. Add the spring onions, if applicable.

4 Stir and cook for a few minutes until warmed through and thickened.

5 Serve with the noodles.

Per serving		% energy
Energy	606 kcal	
Protein	42 g	28%
Fat	18 g	27%
Carbohydrate	73 g	45%
Fibre	5 g	

CHICKEN AND BROCCOLI STIR FRY

You can use any colourful vegetables in this dish, such as mange tout or baby corn.

Makes 4 servings

450 g (1 lb) boneless chicken, skinned and cut into thin strips
1 tbsp oil
2 garlic cloves, chopped
1 in piece root ginger, chopped
450 g (1 lb) broccoli, cut into small florets
1 red pepper, cut into strips
3 tbsp soy sauce
350 g (12 oz) rice or noodles

1 Heat the oil in a wok or heavy-based pan over a high heat.

2 Add the chicken strips, garlic and ginger and stir fry for 2 minutes.

3 Mix in the broccoli and peppers and stir fry for about 5 minutes, until just tender. Add the soy sauce and stir well.

4 Cook the noodles or rice according to directions on the packet and serve with the chicken stir fry.

Per serving		% energy
Energy	543 kcal	
Protein	36 g	26%
Fat	11 g	18%
Carbohydrate	81 g	56%
Fibre	5 g	

RICE AND OTHER GRAINS

139

COUS COUS

Cous cous is made from semolina flour which has been pre-cooked and rolled into tiny clumps. There are three methods of cooking it.

1 Place 600 ml (1 pint) boiling water in a saucepan with a little salt and 350 g (12 oz) cous cous and simmer for 5 minutes.
2 Cover 350 g (12 oz) cous cous with 600 ml (1 pint) boiling water, add a little salt and allow to stand for 15 minutes until all the water has been absorbed.
3 Pour boiling water over the cous cous, allow to stand for a few minutes then transfer to a steamer and steam for 5–6 minutes.

VEGETABLE COUS COUS

Chick peas add protein to this tasty dish

Makes 4 servings

350 g (12 oz) cous cous
600 ml (1 pint) boiling water
1 tbsp olive oil
1 onion, chopped
2 tsp curry powder
450 g (1 lb) vegetables, e.g.
carrots, courgettes, tomatoes, parsnips, green beans, chopped
1 tin (420 g) chick peas
1 vegetable stock cube dissolved in
150 ml (¼ pint) boiling water
50 g (2 oz) chopped dates/50 g
(2 oz) blanched almonds (optional)

1 Cover the cous cous with the boiling water and leave to stand for 15 minutes until all the liquid has been absorbed.

2 Meanwhile, heat the oil in a pan and fry the onion for 5 minutes. Add the curry powder and cook for a further 2 minutes.
3 Add the vegetables, chick peas and stock, bring to the boil, cover and simmer for about 7–10 minutes, or until the vegetables are tender crisp (not soft).
4 Fluff the cous cous with a fork and stir in the dates and almonds, if applicable.
5 Serve topped with the vegetable mixture.

Per serving		% energy
Energy	543 kcal	
Protein	17 g	12%
Fat	7.1 g	13%
Carbohydrate	108 g	75%
Fibre	5.1 g	

BULGAR WHEAT

Bulgar wheat is made from whole wheat which has been cracked, steamed and redried. It requires little or no further cooking and is highly nutritious. You can prepare it in one of two ways.

1. Pour over boiling water (to cover by 2 cm) and leave for approximately 30 minutes to allow the wheat to absorb the water.
2. Boil in a saucepan for approximately 10 minutes.

BULGAR WHEAT PILAFF

Makes 4 servings

1 tbsp olive oil
1 onion, chopped
1 red pepper, chopped
1 garlic clove, crushed
350 g (12 oz) bulgar wheat
900 ml (1½ pints) boiling water
Handful of fresh chopped herbs, e.g. parsley, mint
Lemon juice
Salt and freshly ground black pepper
100 g (4 oz) black olives/175 g (6 oz) diced feta cheese/100 g (4 oz) chopped apricots/100 g (4 oz) toasted cashews, pine nuts or almonds (all optional)

High in B vitamins, iron, magnesium and fibre

1 Heat the olive oil in a pan and cook the onion and pepper for about 5 minutes. Add the garlic and cook for a further 3 minutes.

2 Add the bulgar and boiling water, cover and simmer for 10 minutes until the wheat has absorbed the water and puffed up.

3 Stir in the herbs, any optional ingredients and season with the lemon juice, salt and pepper.

Per serving		% energy
Energy	353 kcal	
Protein	9.1 g	10%
Fat	4.4 g	11%
Carbohydrate	71 g	79%
Fibre	0.9 g	

MILLET

Millet is the seed of a hardy annual grass and is richer in protein and iron than other grains. It is fairly bland on its own but absorbs other flavours well. Use it as an alternative to rice in savoury dishes or in milk puddings.

MILLET PILAFF WITH NUTS AND RAISINS

You can use dried apricots instead of the raisins.

Makes 4 servings

1 tbsp oil
1 large onion, chopped
2 carrots, diced
1 garlic clove, crushed
350 g (12 oz) millet
900 ml (1½ pints) water
Salt and freshly ground black pepper
50 g (2 oz) raisins
50 g (2 oz) toasted flaked almonds

1 Heat the oil in a saucepan and cook the onion for 5 minutes. Add the carrots and garlic and cook for a further 5 minutes.

2 Add the millet and water and season to taste with the salt and pepper. Bring to the boil, cover and simmer for 15–20 minutes, until the water has been absorbed.

3 Stir in the raisins and almonds.

Per serving		% energy
Energy	483 kcal	
Protein	8.9 g	7%
Fat	13 g	24%
Carbohydrate	81 g	69%
Fibre	2.4 g	

15

BEANS AND LENTILS

Don't be put off by the rather cranky image attributed to beans and lentils; they can be used to make many delicious dishes to tempt even the most die-hard 'meat and two veg' person. Many of the following recipes have been inspired by Mexican and Asian cuisines, owing to the subtle spicy flavours and simplicity of cooking. Beans and lentils are among the most nutritious foods, rich in protein, fibre, B vitamins, iron, zinc and calcium. The recipes state tinned varieties to save time, but you may, of course, cook them from dried.

SPICY BEAN ENCHILADAS

This nutritionally balanced dish is one of my firm favourites. Serve with a spinach and watercress salad.

Makes 4 enchiladas

1 tbsp (15 ml) olive oil
1 onion, chopped
2 cloves of garlic, crushed
1 tin (420 g) pinto or red kidney beans (or 175 g/6 oz dried beans, soaked, cooked and drained)
½ tin (200 g) chopped tomatoes
1 tbsp (15 g) taco seasoning mix or 150 g (5 oz) enchilada sauce
4 corn or wheat tortillas
225 g (8 oz) passata with herbs or garlic
50 g (2 oz) grated mature Cheddar cheese
Low fat plain yoghurt, sliced onions, shredded lettuce

1 Heat the oil in a large frying pan. Sauté the onion and garlic for 5 minutes.

2 Add the beans to the pan and mash roughly.

3 Add the tomatoes, taco seasoning (or enchilada sauce) and continue to cook for a few minutes.

4 Spread one quarter of the mixture over each tortilla. Roll up and place seam-side down in a baking dish sprayed with oil spray.

5 Spoon the passata over the tortillas and sprinkle the cheese over the top.

6 Cover with foil and bake at 100°C/350°F/gas mark 4 for 30 minutes. Alternatively, cover and microwave for 7 minutes.

7 Serve with a spoonful of yoghurt, and sprinkle with onions and lettuce.

Per serving		% energy
Energy	328 kcal	
Protein	14 g	17%
Fat	9 g	25%
Carbohydrate	51 g	58%
Fibre	6.9 g	

143

CHICKEN ENCHILADAS

Canned chillis have a milder flavour than fresh. You can of course substitute chopped fresh chillis, according to your taste.

Makes 4 enchiladas

150 g (5 oz) enchilada sauce
225 g (8 oz) tomato salsa
175 g (6 oz) cooked chicken, shredded
50 g (2 oz) canned green chillis, chopped (optional)
4 corn or wheat tortillas
225 g (8 oz) passata
50 g (2 oz) Cheddar cheese, grated
Low fat plain yoghurt, sliced onions, shredded lettuce

1 In a saucepan, combine the enchilada sauce, salsa, chicken and chillis.

2 Bring to the boil, stirring continuously, and simmer for a few minutes.

3 Place one quarter of the chicken mixture on each tortilla and roll up. Place seam-side down in a baking dish sprayed with oil spray.

4 Spoon the passata over the tortillas and sprinkle the cheese over the top.

5 Cover with foil and bake at 180°C/350°F/gas mark 4 for 30 minutes. Alternatively, cover and microwave for 7 minutes.

6 Serve with a spoonful of yoghurt, and sprinkle with onions and lettuce.

Per serving		% energy
Energy	382 kcal	
Protein	23 g	24%
Fat	10 g	24%
Carbohydrate	53 g	52%
Fibre	2.6 g	

STORE-CUPBOARD BEAN BAKE

Ideal as a midweek supper when you are pressed for time, this is one of the speediest dishes that can be assembled from ingredients in the store-cupboard. Use any variety of tinned beans in place of the red kidney beans if you wish.

Quick to make!

Makes 4 servings

1 onion, chopped
1 garlic clove, chopped
2 tsp oil or butter
1 tin (400 g) tomatoes with juice
2 tins (2 × 420 g) red kidney beans, drained
1 tsp mixed herbs
1 vegetable stock cube
40 g (1½ oz) grated Cheddar cheese

1 Heat the oil in a large pan and sauté the onion and garlic over a high heat for 3–4 minutes until golden.

2 Add the tomatoes (roughly broken up), beans, herbs and a crumbled stock cube. Stir well and bring to the boil. Simmer for a few minutes.

3 Spoon into a baking dish and sprinkle with grated cheese.

4 Melt the cheese under a hot grill or microwave for 2 minutes until the cheese is bubbling.

Per serving		% energy
Energy	256 kcal	
Protein	16 g	25%
Fat	6.6 g	23%
Carbohydrate	35 g	52%
Fibre	12 g	

DAHL

This is one of my favourite quick suppers!

Great source of protein, iron, fibre and B vitamins

Makes 4 servings

2 tbsp oil
2 onions, chopped
3–4 garlic cloves, crushed
1 tsp ground cumin
2 tsp ground coriander
1 tsp turmeric
350 g (12 oz) red lentils
1.2 l (2 pints) water
Salt
Chopped fresh coriander, parsley, spring onion (optional)

1 Heat the oil in a large pan and fry the onion for about 5 minutes over a high heat. Add the garlic and spices and fry for a further minute.

2 Add the lentils and water and bring to the boil. Cover and simmer for approximately 20 minutes. Alternatively, cook in a pressure cooker for 3 minutes then turn off the heat.

3 Season with salt to taste and stir in the optional ingredients, if applicable.

Per serving		% energy
Energy	338 kcal	
Protein	21 g	25%
Fat	6.7 g	18%
Carbohydrate	52 g	57%
Fibre	4.7 g	

BEAN AND TOMATO CASSEROLE

This nutritious one-pot meal is simplicity itself. Use any other vegetables (e.g. onions, mushrooms) in place of the leeks if you prefer.

Makes 4 servings

1 tbsp olive oil
2 leeks, sliced
1 tin (400 g) chopped tomatoes
2 tins (2 × 425 g) beans (any variety), drained
1 vegetable stock cube dissolved in 100 ml (4 fl oz) water

1 Heat the oil in a large saucepan. Add the leeks and cook over a moderate to high heat for about 5 minutes until the leeks are soft.

2 Add the remaining ingredients, stir and bring to the boil. Simmer for a further 10–15 minutes, or until the casserole has thickened.

3 Accompany with warm pitta breads.

Per serving		% energy
Energy	204 kcal	
Protein	13 g	25%
Fat	4 g	18%
Carbohydrate	31 g	57%
Fibre	11 g	

BEANS AND LENTILS

145

MEXICAN BEAN BAKE

Perfect for refuelling after exercise, this dish provides complex carbohydrates and protein.

Makes 4 servings

1 onion, chopped
2 cloves garlic, crushed
1 red and 1 green pepper, sliced
1 tsp each of basil and parsley
450 ml (1 pint) passata (sieved tomatoes)
1 vegetable stock cube
1 tin (420 g) red kidney beans, drained
1 tin (420 g) pinto beans, drained
100 g (4 oz) reduced fat mozzarella cheese, sliced

1 Place the onion, garlic, peppers, herbs, passata, stock cube and beans in a large saucepan.
2 Bring to the boil, stirring, and simmer for 10–15 minutes.
3 Spoon the bean mixture into a baking dish then sprinkle over the cheese.
4 Bake uncovered at 200°C/400°F/gas mark 6 for 15 minutes until the cheese is bubbling. Alternatively, microwave for 5 minutes.

Per serving		% energy
Energy	290 kcal	
Protein	24 g	34%
Fat	4.9 g	15%
Carbohydrate	40 g	51%
Fibre	13 g	

TORTILLA STACK

This is a quick, nutritious dish that can be prepared in a few minutes. Serve with a leafy salad.

Makes 4 servings

2 tins (2 × 420 g) pinto beans, drained
1 tin (400 g) sweetcorn, drained
150 g (5 oz) enchilada sauce
8 wheat tortillas
50 g (2 oz) Cheddar cheese, grated
1 sliced beef tomato, sliced onions, salsa (to serve)

1 Place the beans, sweetcorn and enchilada sauce into a large saucepan. Bring to the boil and stir until heated through.
2 Coat a large baking tray with oil spray.
3 Place two tortillas side by side on the tray. Spoon one eighth of the bean mixture onto each tortilla. Sprinkle with about 2 tsp of the cheese.
4 Place another tortilla on top and repeat the layers, finishing with beans and cheese.
5 Loosely cover with foil and bake for 10 minutes at 180°C/350°F/gas mark 4.

Per serving		% energy
Energy	474 kcal	
Protein	24 g	20%
Fat	9.3 g	18%
Carbohydrate	79 g	62%
Fibre	14 g	

ONE-MINUTE BURRITO

Serve with a simple green salad

Makes 1 serving

2 wheat tortillas
½ tin (210 g) refried beans
2 tbsp low fat fromage frais
1 tbsp tomato salsa
Shredded lettuce, sliced tomato

1 Spoon the beans, fromage frais and salsa onto the tortillas.
2 Top with shredded lettuce and tomato then roll up.
3 Warm through in a hot oven for 5 minutes or a microwave for 1 minute.

SPICY BEAN LASAGNE

You can use red kidney beans or tinned green lentils instead of the borlotti beans.

Makes 4 servings

1 onion, chopped
2 tsp olive oil
1 tsp each cumin and coriander
2 tins (2 × 420 g) borlotti beans (or other variety), drained
1 tin (400 g) chopped tomatoes with peppers
12 sheets lasagne (not pre-cook variety)
350 g (12 oz) cottage cheese
40 g (1½ oz) reduced fat mozzarella, grated

1 For the spicy beans, heat the oil in a pan and sauté the onions and spices for 5 minutes.
2 Add the beans and tomatoes, bring to the boil and cook for a few more minutes.
3 Spray a baking dish with oil spray or coat lightly with a little oil.
4 Place 3 sheets of lasagne in the bottom of the dish and cover with one quarter of the beans and one quarter of the cottage cheese. Repeat the layers, finishing with the beans and cottage cheese.
5 Sprinkle with the mozzarella and bake at 180°C/350°F/gas mark 4 for 30 minutes. Alternatively, microwave for 8 minutes, turning the dish twice.

Per serving		% energy
Energy	554 kcal	
Protein	25 g	18%
Fat	3.4 g	6%
Carbohydrate	104 g	76%
Fibre	2.8 g	

Per serving		% energy
Energy	626 kcal	
Protein	39 g	25%
Fat	9.4 g	14%
Carbohydrate	103 g	61%
Fibre	15 g	

BEANS AND LENTILS

BEANS AND LENTILS

MIXED BEAN CHILLI

Serve with rice, tortillas or crusty bread

Makes 4 servings

1 tbsp (15 ml) olive oil
1 large onion, chopped
2–3 garlic cloves, crushed
Pinch of chilli powder, according to your taste
1 tbsp each of tomato purée and paprika
1 tin (420 g) chopped tomatoes
1 tin (420 g) red kidney beans, drained
1 tin (420 g) cannelini beans, drained
500 g (1 lb) mixed vegetables, e.g. carrots, peppers, courgettes

1 Heat the oil in a large pan. Add the onion, garlic and chilli and sauté for 5 minutes.

2 Add the tomato purée and paprika and cook for 2 minutes.

3 Add the tinned tomatoes, beans and vegetables. Stir and bring to the boil. Simmer for 20 minutes, until the vegetables are tender.

4 Serve with cooked rice, tortillas or crusty bread.

Per serving		% energy
Energy	263 kcal	
Protein	14 g	22%
Fat	4.3 g	15%
Carbohydrate	45 g	63%
Fibre	14 g	

SPICY CHICK PEAS WITH TOMATOES

The chick peas provide protein and iron. Serve with cooked rice or pasta.

Makes 4 servings

1 tbsp oil
1 onion, chopped
2 garlic cloves, crushed
1 tin (400 g) chopped tomatoes
1½ tsp curry paste (or according to taste)
2 tins (2 × 420 g) chick peas, drained
150 ml (¼ pint) thick yoghurt
Fresh coriander and mint, if available

1 Heat the oil in a large pan. Add the onion and garlic and fry over a high heat for 5 minutes.

2 Add the tomatoes, curry paste and chick peas. Bring to the boil then simmer for 10 minutes.

3 Stir in the yoghurt and the chopped fresh herbs, if available, just before serving. Do not allow to boil.

Per serving		% energy
Energy	268 kcal	
Protein	16 g	23%
Fat	8.3 g	28%
Carbohydrate	35 g	49%
Fibre	8.1 g	

FISH AND BEAN CASSOULET

This dish is a great source of protein and fibre.

Makes 4 servings

750 g (1½ lb) haddock steaks
1 l (1¾ pints) stock or water
1 bay leaf
1 tbsp oil
1 onion, chopped
2 celery sticks, chopped
2 carrots, chopped
4 tbsp white wine or water
2 tins (2 × 420 g) haricot beans, drained
1 tsp mixed herbs
4 tomatoes, chopped
4 tbsp fresh breadcrumbs
2 tbsp fresh chopped parsley

Balance the meal with a jacket potato

1 Cook the fish in the stock or water with the bay leaf for about 10–15 minutes. Drain, reserving a pint of the liquid.

2 Flake the fish, removing any bones.

3 Heat the oil in a pan and fry the vegetables over a high heat for about 5 minutes.

4 Pour in the reserved fish liquid, wine or extra water, beans and herbs and cook for about 10 minutes, until the liquid has been reduced.

5 Add the cooked fish and tomatoes. Check the seasoning and transfer into a shallow baking dish.

6 Mix the breadcrumbs and parsley together and sprinkle on the top.

7 Bake at 190°C/375°F/gas mark 5 for 30–35 minutes until the top is crisp and golden.

Per serving		% energy
Energy	415 kcal	
Protein	50 g	48%
Fat	5.5 g	12%
Carbohydrate	45 g	40%
Fibre	14 g	

MIXED VEGETABLE AND LENTIL CURRY

Lentils add protein, fibre and iron to the curry. Vary the vegetables according to what you have available.

Makes 4 servings

225 g (8 oz) red lentils
750 ml (1¼ pints) water
2 tbsp olive oil
1 large onion, sliced
1 tsp each of cumin, coriander, turmeric and chilli powder (alternatively use 1 tbsp curry powder)
2 garlic cloves, crushed
900 g (2 lb) vegetables, e.g. cauliflower, courgettes, mushrooms, okra, carrots, tomatoes
Salt

1 Place the lentils and water in a pan and boil for 15 minutes.

2 Heat the oil in a large pan and sauté the onion for 5 minutes.

3 Add the spices and garlic and continue cooking for 2 minutes.

4 Add the vegetables and lentils, bring to the boil, cover and simmer for 10 minutes, or until the vegetables are just tender.

5 Season with salt.

Per serving		% energy
Energy	294 kcal	
Protein	18 g	25%
Fat	7.5 g	23%
Carbohydrate	41 g	52%
Fibre	6.6 g	

BEANS AND LENTILS

149

CHILLI CON CARNE

This is a low fat version of the classic dish, and one which is useful for smuggling extra vegetables into your diet. You may use any type of lean minced meat such as turkey, beef or pork.

Makes 4 servings

350 g (12 oz) lean minced turkey
or beef
1 tbsp oil
1 onion, chopped
2 garlic cloves, crushed
1 green pepper, chopped
2 celery sticks, chopped
1 tbsp paprika
1 tsp chilli powder
1–2 tsp ground cumin
2 tbsp tomato purée
600 ml (1 pint) stock or water
2 tins (2 × 420 g) red kidney beans
350 g (12 oz) rice

1 Dry fry the mince in a non-stick pan for approximately 5 minutes until browned. Drain any fat that separates from the meat. Set aside.

2 Heat the oil in a large pan and sauté the onion, pepper, celery and garlic for 3 minutes. Add the spices and fry for a further minute.

3 Add the tomato purée, stock or water and the beans, cover and simmer for approximately 1 hour (or longer if you wish).

4 Cook the rice according to instructions on the packet and serve with the chilli.

Per serving		% energy
Energy	643 kcal	
Protein	39 g	24%
Fat	9.1 g	13%
Carbohydrate	109 g	63%
Fibre	12 g	

BEAN AND COURGETTE PROVENÇALE WITH GARLIC BREAD

Flageolet beans have a delicate flavour that works really well with tomatoes.

Makes 4 servings

Provençale:
1 tbsp olive oil
2 onions, sliced
2 garlic cloves, crushed
450 g (1 lb) courgettes, sliced
2 tins (2 × 420 g) flageolet beans, drained
1 tin (400 g) tomatoes
1 tsp dried oregano
1 vegetable stock cube dissolved in 150 ml (¼ pint) water
Garlic bread:
1 French stick
40 g (1½ oz) low fat spread
1 garlic clove, crushed

1 Heat the oil in a large pan and sauté the onions for approximately 5 minutes until softened.

2 Add the garlic and courgettes and cook for a further 5 minutes.

3 Add the remaining ingredients. Bring to the boil, cover and simmer for another 10 minutes.

4 To make the garlic bread, slice the stick diagonally at intervals of about 3 cm, almost cutting right through. Mix together the low fat spread and garlic. Spread the mixture in each slit, wrap in foil and bake in a preheated oven at 220°C/425°F/gas mark 7 for 5–10 minutes.

Per serving		% energy
Energy	480 kcal	
Protein	23 g	19%
Fat	10 g	19%
Carbohydrate	79 g	62%
Fibre	14 g	

PASTA 16

Pasta is a perfect food for active people. It has a relatively low glycaemic index which means it produces a gradual, sustained rise in blood sugar levels. It is extremely high in carbohydrate, low in fat and the wholemeal version is a good source of fibre, B vitamins and iron. It is also very quick and easy to cook and can be combined with ready-made or home-made sauces to make a substantial healthy meal.

TOP COOKING TIPS

- Cook pasta in a large pan of fast-boiling water.
- Add a tablespoon of oil to stop the pasta from sticking and the water from boiling over.
- Stir the pasta briefly before partly covering with a lid.
- Cooking time will depend on the shape and thickness of the pasta. Most varieties take between 8–10 minutes; very small pasta takes only 5 minutes. Test a piece by removing from the pan and biting it – it should feel tender yet fairly firm to the bite.
- Drain through a colander.
- Mix the hot pasta with a little olive oil or accompanying sauce.

ATHLETES' HOT PASTA WITH VEGETABLES

Simply add whatever fresh or frozen vegetables you have handy to the pasta pot and – hey presto! Ideal for quick nutritious suppers and attractive enough to serve to guests at dinner. Any left-overs are also good served cold as a salad.

Makes 4 servings

350 g (12 oz) dried pasta of your choice
2 tbsp olive oil or pesto sauce
2 tbsp parmesan, grated
450 g (1 lb) vegetables of your choice (e.g. strips of red, green or yellow peppers, broccoli florets, mushrooms, peas, courgettes)

1 Cook the pasta in plenty of boiling water according to the directions on the packet. Add the vegetables during the last 5 minutes of cooking. Drain.

2 While hot, combine with the olive oil or pesto and parmesan cheese.

3 Stir in the vegetables.

Per serving		% energy
Energy	399 kcal	
Protein	15 g	15%
Fat	9.5 g	21%
Carbohydrate	68 g	64%
Fibre	5.4 g	

Pasta with sauce

Accompany any of the following sauces with your favourite pasta shapes. In general, thin pasta and pasta ribbons (e.g. spaghetti, linguine, tagliatelle) go best with the smoother sauces; pasta shapes (e.g. fussilli, rigatoni, penne, farfelle) go best with chunky sauces containing larger pieces of vegetables or meat. I think pasta sauces are best stirred through the pasta rather than spooned on top. This also avoids the need for added olive oil or butter in the pasta.

As a rough guide, allow approximately 75 g (3 oz) dried pasta per portion. For those with higher carbohydrate needs, 100–150 g (4–5 oz) would be more suitable. For fresh pasta, allow approximately 100 g (4 oz) per portion.

VEGETARIAN BOLOGNESE

Rich in protein, fibre and B vitamins

Makes 4 servings

1 tbsp olive oil
1 onion, chopped
2 carrots, finely chopped
1 large courgette, finely chopped
1 tin (400 g) chopped tomatoes
1 tin (420 g) brown or green lentils (or 100 g (4 oz) dried lentils, soaked and cooked)
1 tsp mixed herbs
1 tbsp parmesan, grated

1 Heat the oil in a large frying pan. Add the vegetables, sauté over a high heat, stirring often until softened (about 5 minutes).
2 Add the tomatoes, lentils and herbs. Bring to the boil, reduce the heat and cook for a few minutes until the sauce thickens slightly.
3 Stir in the cheese and heat through.

Per serving (including 75 g/3 oz dried pasta)		% energy
Energy	467 kcal	
Protein	21 g	18%
Fat	6.1 g	12%
Carbohydrate	87 g	70%
Fibre	7.9 g	

TURKEY BOLOGNESE

Low in fat!

Makes 4 servings

1 tsp olive oil
350 g (12 oz) turkey mince
1 onion, chopped
3 celery stalks, chopped
2 carrots, chopped
1 tin (400 g) chopped tomatoes
2 tbsp tomato purée
1 tsp mixed herbs
Salt and pepper

1 In a large non-stick frying pan, heat the oil. Add the turkey mince and cook, stirring for about 4–5 minutes, until no longer pink.
2 Add the vegetables. Cook for 3–5 minutes, until just tender.
3 Stir in the chopped tomatoes, tomato purée, herbs and seasoning to taste. Heat through.

Per serving (including 75 g/3 oz dried pasta)		% energy
Energy	470 kcal	
Protein	37 g	32%
Fat	5.3 g	10%
Carbohydrate	73 g	58%
Fibre	4.7 g	

PASTA

153

PASTA

A–Z VEGETABLE SAUCE

You can vary this delicious sauce according to what vegetables you have handy.

Makes 4 servings

1 onion, chopped
2 garlic cloves, crushed
1 tin (400 g) chopped tomatoes
2 tbsp tomato purée
2 or more vegetables from the list below*
1 tbsp chopped fresh or 1 tsp dried basil
25 g (1 oz) parmesan, grated

*225 g (8 oz) asparagus, chopped into 4 cm lengths; 2 courgettes, sliced; 1 red, green or yellow pepper, chopped; 225 g (8 oz) broccoli florets; 150 g (5 oz) mange tout; 1 small aubergine, finely chopped; 100 g (4 oz) mushrooms, sliced; 100 g (4oz) peas; 100 g (4 oz) French beans, chopped into 4 cm lengths.

1 Place the onions, garlic and tomatoes in a large non-stick saucepan and boil for 3 minutes, or until the onion is soft.

2 Add the tomato purée, prepared vegetables and basil. Cook for 4 minutes, or until the vegetables are tender but still firm.

3 After combining the sauce with the pasta, sprinkle over the parmesan.

Per serving (including 75 g/3 oz dried pasta)		% energy
Energy	386 kcal	
Protein	18 g	10%
Fat	4.6 g	11%
Carbohydrate	73 g	70%
Fibre	6.2 g	

VEGETARIAN CHILLI SAUCE

Low fat and great for hiding vegetables!

Makes 4 servings

2 tsp olive oil
1 large onion, chopped
2 garlic cloves, crushed
1 small red chilli, deseeded and finely chopped (or ½ tsp dried chilli)
2 celery stalks, finely chopped/
1 green pepper, finely chopped (optional)
1 tin (420 g) red kidney beans, drained
450 ml (1 pint) passata (smooth sieved tomatoes)

1 Heat the oil in a large non-stick pan. Add the onion, garlic and chilli (and the optional vegetables, if applicable) and simmer over a moderate to high heat for 3–4 minutes.

2 Stir in the red kidney beans and passata, bring to the boil and simmer for a few minutes until the sauce has thickened.

Per serving (including 75 g/3 oz dried pasta)		% energy
Energy	428 kcal	
Protein	18 g	17%
Fat	4.2 g	9%
Carbohydrate	85 g	74%
Fibre	9 g	

TOMATO AND TUNA SAUCE

Only 10 minutes to make!

Makes 4 servings

1 onion, chopped
1 garlic clove, crushed
1 tin (400 g) chopped tomatoes
1 tbsp tomato purée
100 g (4 oz) vegetables of choice
(e.g. mushrooms, courgettes)
1 tin (200 g/7 oz) tuna in water or
brine, drained and flaked
1 tsp dried basil

1 Place the onion, garlic and tomatoes
   in a large non-stick frying pan and
   sauté for 4–5 minutes until the
   onion is soft.
2 Stir in the tomato purée and
   vegetables and cook for 5 minutes.
3 Add the tuna and basil and heat
   through.

Per serving (including 75 g/3 oz dried pasta)		% energy
Energy	369 kcal	
Protein	22 g	24%
Fat	2.2 g	5%
Carbohydrate	70 g	71%
Fibre	3.9 g	

QUICK TUNA AND SWEETCORN SAUCE

You can add other ingredients, such as frozen peas, mushrooms or chopped peppers to the sauce.

Ready in five minutes!

Makes 4 servings

1 jar (400 g) ready-made pasta
sauce (any variety)
1 tin (225 g) sweetcorn, drained
1 tin (200 g) tuna in water or
brine, drained and flaked

1 Place the pasta sauce, sweetcorn
   and tuna in a saucepan, bring to the
   boil and cook for 3–4 minutes, until
   well heated through.

Per serving (including 75 g/3 oz dried pasta)		% energy
Energy	480 kcal	
Protein	26 g	22%
Fat	6.4 g	12%
Carbohydrate	84 g	66%
Fibre	4.5 g	

PASTA

TOMATO AND HERB SAUCE

You can substitute passata (smooth sieved tomatoes) for the tinned tomatoes.

Makes 4 servings

2 tsp olive oil
I onion, chopped
2 garlic cloves, crushed
I red and I green pepper, chopped
I tin (400 g) chopped tomatoes
I tbsp each of fresh basil, fresh parsley and fresh chives (alternatively, use I tbsp dried mixed herbs)

I Heat the oil in a large frying pan. Add the onion and garlic and cook for 3 minutes.
2 Add the peppers and cook for 3–4 minutes, until softened.
3 Add the tinned tomatoes and heat through or, time permitting, simmer for 5 minutes.
4 Stir in the herbs just before serving.

CHEESE SAUCE

This low fat cheese sauce tastes as creamy and rich as the traditional version and is easy to make too.

Makes 4 servings

600 ml (I pint) skimmed or semi-skimmed milk
2 level tbsp cornflour
½ tsp Dijon mustard
75 g (3 oz) extra mature Cheddar cheese, grated
Freshly ground black pepper

I Blend the cornflour with a little of the milk in a jug. Gradually add the remainder of the milk, stirring constantly.
2 Pour into a saucepan and heat, stirring constantly until the sauce just reaches the boil and has thickened.
3 Remove from the heat, stir in the mustard, cheese and freshly ground black pepper to taste. Serve immediately to prevent a skin forming over the surface.

Per serving (including 75 g/3 oz dried pasta)		% energy
Energy	355 kcal	
Protein	12 g	14%
Fat	3.9 g	10%
Carbohydrate	72 g	76%
Fibre	4.8 g	

Per serving (including 75 g/3 oz dried pasta)		% energy
Energy	463 kcal	
Protein	21 g	18%
Fat	9.1 g	18%
Carbohydrate	79 g	64%
Fibre	2.6 g	

HAM AND MUSHROOM SAUCE

You can use lean back bacon instead of the ham.

Makes 4 servings

1 tsp olive oil
4 slices (100 g) ham (preferably reduced salt), chopped
225 g (8 oz) small mushrooms, halved
2 tbsp cornflour
600 ml (1 pint) skimmed or semi-skimmed milk
1 tsp dried oregano or basil
Freshly ground black pepper

1 Heat the oil in a large frying pan. Sauté the ham and mushrooms for 4–5 minutes.
2 Stir in the cornflour together with a little milk. Gradually add the rest of the milk, stirring continuously.
3 Heat until the sauce just reaches boiling point. Remove from the heat and stir in the herbs and pepper.

Per serving (including 75 g/3 oz dried pasta)		% energy
Energy	429 kcal	
Protein	22 g	21%
Fat	4.7 g	10%
Carbohydrate	79 g	69%
Fibre	3.2 g	

CHICKEN AND MUSHROOM SAUCE

Add any vegetables you have to the sauce, such as chopped peppers or spring onions.

Makes 4 servings

1 tbsp oil
1 onion, chopped
4 boneless chicken breasts (approx. 75 g/3 oz each), sliced into 1 cm strips
100 g (4 oz) mushrooms, sliced
225 g (8 oz) low fat crème fraîche
Juice of ½ lemon
Freshly ground black pepper

1 Heat the oil in a non-stick frying pan. Cook the onion over a high to moderate heat for 3–4 minutes until softened.
2 Add the chicken strips and cook for 3 minutes.
3 Stir in the mushrooms followed by the crème fraîche, lemon juice and black pepper to taste. Cook for 2–3 minutes until well heated through.

Per serving (including 75 g/3 oz dried pasta)		% energy
Energy	465 kcal	
Protein	34 g	29%
Fat	7.3 g	14%
Carbohydrate	70 g	57%
Fibre	3.1 g	

PASTA

157

BASIC RED LENTIL SAUCE

A good source of protein, fibre and minerals

Makes 4 servings

2 tsp oil
I onion, chopped
2 garlic cloves, crushed
225 g (8 oz) red lentils
800 ml (1½ pints) water
2 vegetable stock cubes or 3 tsp
Swiss Vegetable Bouillon
I red, yellow or green pepper/2
courgettes/2 carrots/100 g (4 oz)
mushrooms/I small aubergine
(all optional)

I Heat the oil in a large non-stick
saucepan or pressure cooker. Sauté
the onion and garlic for 3–4
minutes.

2 Add the lentils, water and stock
cubes or concentrate.

3 Bring to the boil, stirring to dissolve
the stock. Simmer for 30 minutes or
cook in the pressure cooker for 3
minutes then remove from the heat.

4 Add optional vegetables of your
choice and continue to cook for a
further 10 minutes until the
vegetables are tender.

Per serving (including 75 g/3 oz dried pasta)		% energy
Energy	502 kcal	
Protein	24 g	19%
Fat	4.3 g	8%
Carbohydrate	98 g	73%
Fibre	5.5 g	

PASTA ONE-POT DISHES

PASTA AND LENTIL POT

*This delicious vegetarian dish is perfectly
nutritionally balanced for athletes.*

Makes 4 servings

350 g (12 oz) fusilli
2 large carrots, thinly sliced
100 g (4 oz) frozen peas
I tbsp olive oil
I onion, chopped
I clove garlic, crushed
I can (400 g) lentil soup
15 g (½ oz) parmesan cheese,
grated

I Boil the fusilli in a large saucepan of
water for about 5 minutes. Add the
carrots and continue cooking for a
further 3 minutes. Add the peas and
cook for a further 2 minutes. Drain.

2 Meanwhile, sauté the onion and
garlic in the olive oil until soft. Add
to the fusilli.

3 Add the soup to the pasta pot and
cook until hot, about 2 minutes. Stir
in the parmesan cheese and serve.

Per serving		% energy
Energy	476 kcal	
Protein	19 g	16%
Fat	10 g	19%
Carbohydrate	84 g	65%
Fibre	6.4 g	

BAKED MACARONI PIE

Great dish for adding extra vegetables to your diet!

Makes 4 servings

1 tsp olive oil
1 large onion, sliced
225 g (8 oz) sliced vegetables of your choice, e.g. mushrooms, peppers, tomatoes, courgettes
2 tbsp low fat spread
2 tbsp cornflour
600 ml (1 pint) skimmed milk
50 g (2 oz) mature Cheddar cheese
350 g (12 oz) macaroni

1 In a non-stick pan, sauté the vegetables in the olive oil over a high heat until browned.
2 Whisk together the low fat spread, cornflour and milk in a saucepan over a medium heat until thickened. Stir in the cheese.
3 Boil the macaroni in a large saucepan for 10 minutes. Drain.
4 In a large pyrex baking dish, layer half the macaroni, vegetables and sauce and repeat, finishing with a layer of sauce.
5 Bake in an oven at 180°C/350°F/gas mark 4 until hot and bubbly (about 20 minutes). Alternatively, cook in a microwave at full power for 7 minutes.

Per serving		% energy
Energy	495 kcal	
Protein	21 g	17%
Fat	10 g	19%
Carbohydrate	85 g	64%
Fibre	8.5 g	

TUNA AND PASTA BAKE

Add any vegetables you have available – such as frozen peas or green beans.

Makes 4 servings

Pasta bake:
2 tsp olive oil
1 onion, sliced
3 sticks of celery, chopped
100 g (4 oz) mushrooms, sliced
350 g (12 oz) dry weight pasta shells, cooked
3 tbsp fresh parsley, chopped
1 tin (200 g/7 oz) tuna in water or brine, drained
White sauce:
1 tbsp low fat spread
1 tbsp cornflour
450 ml (¾ pint) skimmed milk

1 In a non-stick frying pan, sauté the vegetables in the olive oil over a moderate heat.
2 Prepare the white sauce by whisking all the sauce ingredients in a pan over a medium heat until thickened.
3 Spoon layers of the vegetables, pasta, tuna and white sauce into a baking dish, sprinkling parsley between each layer and finishing with a layer of the sauce.
4 Bake at 190°C/375°F/gas mark 5 for 20 minutes. Alternatively cook in the microwave for 6 minutes.

Per serving		% energy
Energy	437 kcal	
Protein	26 g	24%
Fat	5.6 g	11%
Carbohydrate	76 g	65%
Fibre	3.5 g	

PASTA

PASTA WITH SPINACH AND CHEESE

Makes 4 servings

350 g (12 oz) dried ribbon pasta, e.g. tagliatelle
1 tbsp oil
2 garlic cloves, crushed
450 g (1 lb) fresh or frozen spinach
½ tsp nutmeg
100 g (4 oz) fromage blanc or low fat soft cheese
Salt and freshly ground black pepper

Spinach is an excellent source of iron, folic acid and vitamin C

1 Cook the pasta in boiling water according to directions on the packet. Drain.
2 Meanwhile, heat the oil in a frying pan and sauté the garlic for 2 minutes over a moderate heat.
3 Add the spinach and stir until the spinach is wilted, about 2 minutes.
4 Add the nutmeg and quark or low fat soft cheese. Combine well and heat through.
5 Add the drained pasta and season to taste.

Per serving		% energy
Energy	370 kcal	
Protein	16 g	17%
Fat	5.3 g	13%
Carbohydrate	69 g	70%
Fibre	4.9 g	

PASTA WITH BEANS

Makes 4 servings

350 g (12 oz) pasta shapes
1 jar (400 g) ready made pasta sauce
1 tin (420 g) beans*
2 tbsp parmesan, grated

Only 10 minutes to make!

1 Cook the pasta in boiling water according to directions on the packet. Drain.
2 Meanwhile, combine the pasta sauce and beans in a saucepan and heat through.
3 Add the drained pasta. Serve topped with the parmesan.

*This recipe works well with chick peas, red kidney beans, or pinto beans.

Per serving		% energy
Energy	493 kcal	
Protein	22 g	18%
Fat	8.6 g	16%
Carbohydrate	87 g	66%
Fibre	6.8 g	

PASTA WITH CHEESE AND WALNUTS

This may sound like an odd combination if you've never tried it before, but it is one which works surprisingly well. This is an adapted version of my mother's Hungarian recipe.

Walnuts are a great source of omega-3 fatty acids

Makes 4 servings

350 g (12 oz) tagliatelle or other ribbon pasta
50 g (2 oz) chopped or roughly crushed walnuts
225 g (8 oz) cottage cheese
2 tsp brown sugar

1 Cook the pasta according to directions on the packet. Drain.

2 Combine the walnuts, cottage cheese and sugar.

3 Stir in the pasta and heat through (do not overheat).

MEAT LASAGNE (LOW FAT VERSION)

Add other vegetables, e.g. mushrooms, peppers, spinach, to the mince mixture instead of the courgettes, depending on what you have available.

Makes 4 servings

1 onion, chopped
2 courgettes, sliced
225 g (8 oz) extra lean beef mince (or turkey mince)
1 tin (400 g) chopped tomatoes
3 tbsp tomato purée
1 tsp basil or oregano
Salt and pepper to taste
12 sheets lasagne (not pre-cook variety)
350 g (12 oz) cottage cheese
75 g (3 oz) reduced fat mozzarella

1 Heat a large non-stick frying pan. Cook the onion, courgette and mince, stirring frequently, for 5–6 minutes until the mince is no longer pink. Drain off any fat.

2 Add the tomatoes, tomato purée, and herbs. Season with salt and pepper to taste.

3 Place 4 sheets of lasagne at the bottom of an oiled baking dish. Spoon over one third of the meat mixture and one third of the cottage cheese.

4 Repeat the layers, finishing with a layer of cottage cheese.

5 Cover with very thin slices of mozzarella.

6 Bake at 180°C/350°F/gas mark 4 for 30 minutes.

Per serving		% energy
Energy	467 kcal	
Protein	20 g	18%
Fat	4 g	27%
Carbohydrate	69 g	55%
Fibre	3.1 g	

Per serving		% energy
Energy	548 kcal	
Protein	44 g	32%
Fat	10 g	17%
Carbohydrate	75 g	51%
Fibre	4.5 g	

PASTA

BEAN LASAGNE

The red kidney beans in this dish add protein and extra fibre. You can also make it with butter beans or pinto beans.

Makes 4 servings

1 tbsp olive oil
1 onion
225 g (8 oz) vegetables of your choice*
1 tbsp taco seasoning mix (or mild curry powder)
1 tin (400 g) red kidney beans, drained
400 g (14 oz) passata (smooth sieved tomatoes)
225 g (8 oz) low fat fromage frais
40 g (1½ oz) mature Cheddar cheese, grated
12 sheets lasagne (pre-cooked variety)

1 Heat the oil in a large frying pan. Cook the onion for 3–4 minutes over a moderate heat. Add the vegetables and continue cooking for 2–3 minutes.

2 Stir in the taco seasoning or curry powder, beans and passata. Simmer for a few minutes until the sauce thickens slightly.

3 Lay 4 sheets of lasagne at the bottom of an oiled baking dish. Cover with one third of the bean mixture. Continue with the layers, finishing with the bean mixture.

4 Spoon over the fromage frais and sprinkle with the cheese.

5 Bake at 180°C/350°F/gas mark 4 for 30 minutes.

* e.g. broccoli florets, green beans, courgettes, peppers.

Per serving		% energy
Energy	530 kcal	
Protein	27 g	20%
Fat	9.3 g	16%
Carbohydrate	91 g	64%
Fibre	11 g	

CHICKEN AND MUSHROOMS WITH PASTA

To balance the meal, serve with a leafy salad

Makes 4 servings

4 chicken drumsticks or thighs, skinned
1 tbsp olive oil
1 onion, sliced
2 green or red peppers, sliced
225 g (8 oz) mushrooms, sliced
450 ml (16 fl oz) passata (smooth sieved tomatoes)
350 g (12 oz) small pasta shapes
300 ml (½ pint) stock or water

1 Sauté the chicken drumsticks in the oil over a high heat until it is browned. Remove from the pan and set aside on a plate.

2 Add the onions, peppers and mushrooms to the pan and cook for 5–10 minutes over a moderate heat.

3 Add the passata, chicken, pasta and stock or water. Bring to the boil and simmer until the pasta is tender and the chicken cooked through, about 10 minutes.

4 Accompany with warm French bread.

Per serving		% energy
Energy	470 kcal	
Protein	31 g	26%
Fat	8.6 g	17%
Carbohydrate	72 g	57%
Fibre	5.4 g	

PASTA 'N' PEAS

This is one of my favourite emergency meals if I'm pressed for time and the store cupboard is nearly empty. It takes 10 minutes to make and is a near-perfect nutritionally balanced meal.

Makes 4 servings

350 g (12 oz) pasta shapes
225 g (8 oz) frozen peas
250 ml (9 fl oz) passata (smooth sieved tomatoes)
Salt and freshly ground
black pepper
1 tsp dried oregano
1–2 tbsp grated parmesan

1 Cook the pasta in boiling water for 7 minutes. Add the peas and continue cooking for a further 3 minutes. Drain.

2 Stir in the passata, salt, pepper, oregano and parmesan. Heat through then serve.

Per serving		% energy
Energy	359 kcal	
Protein	15 g	17%
Fat	3 g	7%
Carbohydrate	72 g	76%
Fibre	5.8 g	

PASTA

17 BREAD

Home-made bread is surprisingly easy to make, and good exercise for the forearms and shoulders! The effort is truly worth it as it tastes entirely different from mass-produced sliced bread. Don't be put off by the length of time it takes to make – go and have a workout while the dough rises!

BASIC BROWN BREAD

Using a half wholemeal, half white flour mixture produces a lighter bread than 100% wholemeal.

Makes 2 loaves (12 slices each)

225 g (8 oz) strong white flour
225 g (8 oz) strong wholemeal flour
1 sachet easy blend yeast
1½ tsp salt
350 ml (12 fl oz) warm water (or half water, half milk)
1 tbsp oil

1 Mix together the flours, yeast and salt in a large bowl.

2 Make a well in the centre and add the oil and half of the water (or milk). Stir with a wooden spoon, gradually adding more liquid until you have a pliable dough.

3 Turn the dough out onto a floured surface. Knead, adding a little more flour if necessary, until you have a smooth, elastic, not-too-sticky dough. This should take 5–10 minutes.

4 Place the dough in a clean lightly-oiled bowl, cover with a tea towel and leave in a warm place for approximately 1 hour, or until doubled in size.

5 Punch down the dough and knead for a further 5 minutes.

6 Shape into 2 loaves and place in lightly-oiled tins or on a baking sheet. Make 3 or 4 shallow cuts with a knife, cover with a tea towel, and leave for 30 minutes until almost doubled in size.

7 Brush with milk and bake at 200°C/400°F/gas mark 6 for 40–50 minutes. The loaves should sound hollow when tapped on the bottom.

Variations

• White Bread: replace the wholemeal flour with white. You will need a little less liquid.

• Bread Rolls: after the first rising, roll the dough into balls. Reduce the baking time to 30–35 minutes.

• Herb Bread: add 2 tsp dried mixed herbs to the flour mixture.

• Italian Bread: add 2 tbsp olive oil and 2 tsp dried oregano or rosemary to the mixture. Shape into 2 flat rounds and brush with a little olive oil instead of milk.

• Oatmeal Bread: replace 100 g (4 oz) of the wholemeal flour with 100 g (4 oz) oatmeal.

Per serving (1 slice)		% energy
Energy	65 kcal	
Protein	2.3 g	14%
Fat	0.8 g	11%
Carbohydrate	13 g	75%
Fibre	1.1 g	

SODA BREAD

This recipe uses baking powder instead of yeast to make the bread rise, and also requires no kneading so it really is a super-quick method of making your own nutritious bread. The texture is between that of a bread and a cake – it is light, crumbly and definitely moreish. It only keeps fresh for two days but chances are there won't be anything left after a day!

Makes 1 loaf (12 slices)

100 g (4 oz) wholemeal flour
100 g (4 oz) white flour
1 tbsp baking powder
½ tsp salt
2 cartons (2 × 125 g) plain yoghurt
200 ml (7 fl oz) skimmed milk
1 level tbsp honey

1 Mix together the flours, baking powder and salt in a bowl. Make a well in the centre.

2 Mix together the yoghurt, milk and honey in a separate bowl.

3 Pour this liquid mixture into the centre of the dry ingredients. Mix with a wooden spoon until thoroughly blended. The dough should be very soft, almost like a stiff cake batter. Add a little more milk or flour if necessary.

4 With your floured hands, form into a round loaf (or your preferred shape) and place on a lightly-oiled baking tray. Cut a shallow cross on the top.

5 Bake at 200°C/400°F/gas mark 6 for approximately 35 minutes. The loaf should sound hollow when tapped on the bottom.

Variations

- Cheese Soda Bread: add 50 g (2 oz) grated mature cheese to the dry ingredients.
- Nutty Soda Bread: add 75 g (3 oz) chopped walnuts, pecans or almonds to the dry ingredients.
- Herb Soda Bread: add ½ tsp each of dried basil, tarragon, parsley and thyme to the dry ingredients.

CORNMEAL BREAD

This recipe also uses baking powder to raise the bread and produces a fantastically light, cake-like result. It is particularly good served with soups, stews, hot pots and any Mexican dish. Cornmeal has a higher fibre and vitamin content than white flour.

Makes 1 loaf (16 slices)

100 g (4 oz) white or wholemeal flour
100 g (4 oz) yellow cornmeal
1 tbsp baking powder
¼ tsp salt
1 tbsp honey or sugar
1 egg
2 cartons (2 × 125 g) plain yoghurt or 250 ml buttermilk
50 g (2 oz) chopped canned green chillies*/1 can (112 g) creamed sweetcorn/½ tsp chilli powder/ 50 g (2 oz) grated cheese (all optional)

*Canned chillis are less hot than fresh chillis. Feel free to use chopped fresh chillis, according to your taste.

1 Mix together the flour, cornmeal, baking powder and salt in a bowl.

2 Make a well in the centre.

3 Mix together the honey or sugar, egg and yoghurt or buttermilk. Pour this into the well together with any optional ingredients.

4 Mix together briefly with a wooden spoon (do not overmix). This should produce a soft cake-like batter.

5 Spread into an oiled 20 cm (8 in) square baking dish. Bake at 190°C/ 375°F/gas mark 5 for 30–35 minutes.

Per serving (1 slice)		% energy
Energy	90 kcal	
Protein	3.9 g	18%
Fat	0.6 g	5%
Carbohydrate	18 g	77%
Fibre	1.3 g	

Per serving (1 slice)		% energy
Energy	73 kcal	
Protein	2.6 g	15%
Fat	0.9 g	11%
Carbohydrate	14 g	74%
Fibre	0.4 g	

RAISIN BREAD

This bread is high in complex carbohy-drate, low in fat and the raisins add subtle sweetness and extra fibre.

Perfect snack for eating on the run!

Makes I loaf (16 slices)

225 g (8 oz) flour (half wholemeal, half white)
I tbsp baking powder
½ tsp salt
3 tbsp oil
I egg
250 ml (8 fl oz) skimmed milk
I tbsp honey
100 g (4 oz) raisins

1 Mix together the flour, baking powder and salt in a bowl. Make a well in the centre.
2 Mix together the egg, milk and honey in a separate bowl.
3 Pour this liquid mixture into the centre of the dry ingredients together with the raisins. Mix with a wooden spoon until thoroughly blended. The batter should be very soft, almost like a stiff cake batter.
4 Spoon into an oiled 20 cm (8 in) round cake tin or small loaf tin.
5 Bake at 190°C/375°F/gas mark 5 for 30–35 minutes until lightly browned on top. It should sound hollow when tapped on the bottom.

Per serving (I slice)		% energy
Energy	100 kcal	
Protein	2.7 g	11%
Fat	2.8 g	25%
Carbohydrate	17 g	64%
Fibre	I g	

FOCACCIA BREAD

This is a large flat Italian bread, flavoured with olive oil, salt, garlic or herbs.

Makes 2 focaccia (8 slices each)

450 g (I lb) strong white flour
I sachet easy blend yeast
I tsp salt
325 ml (II fl oz) warm water
3 tbsp olive oil
12 black olives/3–4 chopped cloves garlic/2 tbsp chopped fresh rosemary (all optional)

1 Mix the flour, yeast, salt in a large bowl.
2 Make a well in the centre and add I tbsp each of oil and water. Stir with a wooden spoon until you have a soft dough.
3 Turn the dough out onto a floured surface. Knead into a smooth dough – add a little flour if necessary. This should take 5–10 mins.
4 Place the dough in a lightly-oiled bowl, cover with a tea towel and leave in a warm place for I hour/ until doubled in size.
5 Punch down the dough, knead briefly, halve and roll into 2 round or oval shapes.
6 Brush the surface with a little olive oil, cover with a tea towel, and leave for approx. 30 mins.
7 Using your fingertips, dimple the surface of the dough, pushing about halfway in. Brush with the remaining oil and scatter over any optional ingredients. Bake at 200°C/400°F/gas mark 6 for 25 minutes, or until golden.

Per serving (I slice)		% energy
Energy	114 kcal	
Protein	3.2 g	11%
Fat	2.5 g	19%
Carbohydrate	21 g	70%
Fibre	0.9 g	

BREAD

HERB FLATBREAD

The perfect bread for eating with Italian food, main course salads, grilled vegetables and grilled chicken dishes.

Makes I loaf (8 slices)

225 g (8 oz) strong white flour
½ tsp salt
I tbsp olive oil
½ sachet easy blend yeast
175 ml (6 fl oz) warm water or milk
2 tbsp fresh chopped herbs, e.g. oregano, rosemary, thyme

1 Mix together the flour, salt, olive oil and yeast in a large bowl.
2 Make a well in the middle and slowly add the warm water or milk, mixing with a large wooden spoon until the dough comes together.
3 Turn out onto a floured surface and knead until you have a smooth elastic dough.
4 Place in an oiled bowl, cover and leave in a warm place for approximately I hour, until the dough is doubled in volume.

5 Punch the dough down. Knead a few times while incorporating the herbs.
6 Shape into a large flat round loaf, about 30 cm (12 in) in diameter. Brush with a little olive oil. Place on a baking tray, and leave to rise in a warm place for a further 20–30 minutes. Bake at 200°C/400°F/gas mark 6 for about 25 minutes until golden.

Variations

• Cheese and Onion Flatbread: substitute I small finely chopped onion for the herbs. Sprinkle a little Cheddar over the top just before baking.
• Sun-dried Tomato Flatbread: add 75 g (3 oz) chopped sun-dried tomatoes (drained) and sprinkle the top with parmesan just before baking.

Per serving (I slice)		% energy
Energy	109 kcal	
Protein	3.3 g	12%
Fat	1.8 g	15%
Carbohydrate	21 g	73%
Fibre	0.9 g	

BREAD

169

OATMEAL BREAD

A terrific loaf that's perfect with a chunk of cheese or spread with honey at breakfast. Oats add extra fibre (soluble), B vitamins and protein.

Makes I loaf (16 slices)

225 g (8 oz) strong white flour
100 g (4 oz) oats
1½ tsp salt
1 sachet yeast
2 tbsp sugar
4 tbsp margarine or butter
250 ml (8 fl oz) warm water

1 Mix together the flour, oats, salt, yeast and sugar in a large bowl. Rub in the margarine or butter.

2 Make a well in the middle and slowly add the warm water, mixing with a wooden spoon until the dough comes together.

3 Turn out onto a floured surface and knead until you have a smooth elastic dough.

4 Place in an oiled bowl, cover and leave in a warm place for approximately 1 hour, until the dough is doubled in volume.

5 Punch the dough down. Knead for a few more minutes.

6 Shape into an oval or round loaf. Place on a baking tray, leave to rise in a warm place for a further 30 minutes and brush with a little milk. Sprinkle with some extra oats and bake at 200°C/400°F/gas mark 6 for about 25 minutes until golden.

Variations

- Cinnamon Oatmeal Bread: add ½ tsp cinnamon to the flour mixture.

- Honey Nut Oatmeal Bread: substitute honey for the sugar. Incorporate 100 g (4 oz) chopped walnuts during the second kneading.

Per serving (1 slice)		% energy
Energy	105 kcal	
Protein	2.6 g	10%
Fat	3 g	25%
Carbohydrate	18 g	65%
Fibre	1 g	

SUNFLOWER BREAD

This bread has a wonderful nutty taste and a slightly crumbly texture. The sunflower seeds are rich in vitamin E, essential fatty acids and protein (substitute pumpkin seeds if you prefer).

Makes I loaf (16 slices)

100 g (4 oz) strong wholemeal flour
175 g (6 oz) strong white flour
50 g (2 oz) oats
¾ tsp salt
1 sachet easy blend yeast
250 ml (8 fl oz) warm water
2 tbsp oil
2 tbsp honey
50 g (2 oz) sunflower seeds

1 Mix together the flours, oats, salt, and yeast in a large bowl.

2 Mix together the water, oil and honey. Make a well in the middle of the flour and slowly add the liquid until the dough comes together.

3 Turn out onto a floured surface and knead until you have a smooth elastic dough.

4 Place in an oiled bowl, cover and leave in a warm place for approximately 1 hour, until the dough is doubled in volume.

5 Punch the dough down. Knead for a few more minutes, incorporating the sunflower seeds (reserve 1 tablespoonful).

6 Place in a 2 lb loaf tin, leave to rise in a warm place for a further 30 minutes and brush with a little milk.

Sprinkle with the reserved sunflower seeds. Bake at 200°C/400°F/gas mark 6 for 30–40 minutes until firm and golden.

Per serving (I slice)		% energy
Energy	118 kcal	
Protein	3.5 g	12%
Fat	3.8 g	29%
Carbohydrate	19 g	59%
Fibre	1.5 g	

BANANA BREAD

Spread with a little butter, this slightly sweet bread is the perfect refuelling snack.

Makes I loaf (16 slices)

225 g (8 oz) strong white flour
100 g (4 oz) oats
1 tsp salt
1 sachet easy blend yeast
1 tbsp honey or sugar
2 tbsp oil
150 ml (5 fl oz) warm water
2 large bananas, mashed

1 Mix together the flour, oats, salt, yeast and honey or sugar in a large bowl.

2 Mix the oil and water. Make a well in the middle and slowly add the liquid and mashed bananas, mixing with a wooden spoon until the dough comes together.

3 Turn out onto a floured surface and knead until you have a smooth elastic dough.

4 Place in an oiled bowl, cover and leave in a warm place for approximately 1 hour, until the dough is doubled in volume.

5 Punch the dough down. Knead for a few more minutes.

6 Place in a 2 lb loaf tin, leave to rise in a warm place for a further 30 minutes and brush with a little milk. Bake at 200°C/400°F/gas mark 6 for 30–40 minutes until golden.

Per serving (I slice)		% energy
Energy	109 kcal	
Protein	2.8 g	10%
Fat	2.3 g	19%
Carbohydrate	21 g	71%
Fibre	1.1 g	

BREAD

BLUEBERRY BREAD

This is one of my favourites: it's slightly sweet with a light cake-like texture. If you don't have blueberries, substitute raisins.

Makes 1 loaf (16 slices)
100 g (4 oz) cornmeal
225 g (8 oz) strong white flour
1½ tsp salt
1 sachet easy blend yeast
2 tbsp sugar
175 g (6 oz) cottage cheese
1½ tbsp butter or margarine
75 ml (3 fl oz) warm water
175 g (6 oz) fresh blueberries (or 75 g/3 oz dried)

1 Mix together the cornmeal, flour, salt, yeast and sugar in a large bowl.
2 Mix in the cottage cheese and butter or margarine using a fork. Make a well in the middle and slowly add the water until the dough comes together.
3 Turn out onto a floured surface and knead until you have a smooth elastic dough.
4 Place in an oiled bowl, cover and leave in a warm place for approximately 1 hour, until the dough is doubled in volume.
5 Punch the dough down. Knead for a few more minutes, incorporating the blueberries.
6 Place in a 2 lb loaf tin, leave to rise in a warm place for a further 30 minutes and brush with a little milk. Bake at 200°C/400°F/gas mark 6 for 30–40 minutes until firm and golden.

Per serving (1 slice)		% energy
Energy	105 kcal	
Protein	4 g	15%
Fat	1.7 g	14%
Carbohydrate	19 g	71%
Fibre	1 g	

COCONUT PINEAPPLE BREAD

A wonderful fun bread; great for Sunday brunch or for an afternoon snack.

Makes 1 loaf (16 slices)
225 g (8 oz) strong white flour
⅔ tsp salt
1 sachet easy blend yeast
2 tbsp sugar
2½ tbsp grated coconut (or desiccated)
2½ tbsp oil
2–3 tbsp milk
175 g (6 oz) fromage frais
175 g (6 oz) tinned crushed pineapple, drained

1 Mix together the flour, salt, yeast, sugar and coconut in a large bowl.
2 Add the oil, milk, fromage frais and pineapple and mix using a fork.
3 Turn out onto a floured surface and knead until you have a smooth elastic dough.
4 Place in an oiled bowl, cover and leave in a warm place for approximately 1 hour, until the dough is doubled in volume.
5 Punch the dough down. Knead for a few more minutes.
6 Place in a 2 lb loaf tin, leave to rise in a warm place for a further 30 minutes and brush with a little milk. Bake at 200°C/400°F/gas mark 6 for 30–40 minutes until firm and golden.

Per serving (1 loaf)		% energy
Energy	92 kcal	
Protein	2.6 g	12%
Fat	2.9 g	28%
Carbohydrate	15 g	60%
Fibre	0.7 g	

ORANGE CINNAMON BREAD

Excellent for boosting your energy levels in the morning.

Makes 1 loaf (12 slices)

225 g (8 oz) strong white flour
½ tsp salt
1 sachet easy blend yeast
1 tsp sugar
1½ tsp cinnamon
1 tsp grated orange peel
1½ tbsp butter or margarine
175 ml (6 fl oz) orange juice

1 Mix together the flour, salt, yeast, sugar, cinnamon and orange peel in a large bowl. Rub in the butter or margarine.
2 Slowly add the orange juice until the dough comes together.
3 Turn out onto a floured surface and knead until you have a smooth elastic dough.
4 Place in an oiled bowl, cover and leave in a warm place for approximately 1 hour, until the dough is doubled in volume.
5 Punch the dough down. Knead for a few more minutes.
6 Place in a 2 lb loaf tin, leave to rise in a warm place for a further 30 minutes and brush with a little milk. Bake at 200°C/400°F/gas mark 6 for 30–40 minutes, until firm and golden.

Per serving (1 slice)		% energy
Energy	80 kcal	
Protein	2.2 g	11%
Fat	1.3 g	15%
Carbohydrate	16 g	74%
Fibre	0.6 g	

FRUIT BUNS

Make a large batch for the freezer. They are a convenient snack for post-workout refuelling or even breakfast on the run.

Makes 12 servings

350 g (12 oz) strong white flour
½ tsp salt
1 sachet easy blend yeast
40 g (1½ oz) sugar
1 tsp cinnamon
175 ml (6 fl oz) milk
2 eggs
3 tbsp butter or margarine, melted
100 g (4 oz) raisins

1 Mix together the flour, salt, yeast, sugar and cinnamon in a large bowl.
2 Mix together the milk, eggs and melted butter in a separate bowl. Make a well in the flour and gradually add the liquid, stirring until the dough comes together.
3 Turn out onto a floured surface and knead into a smooth elastic dough.
4 Place in an oiled bowl, cover and leave in a warm place for approx. 1 hour, until the dough is doubled in volume.
5 Punch the dough down. Knead for a few more minutes, incorporating the raisins.
6 Cut the dough into 12 equal pieces, shape into balls and place on an oiled baking tray. Cover and leave to rise in a warm place for approx. 30 mins or until doubled in volume. Brush with milk and bake at 190°C/375°F/gas mark 5 for 20–25 mins.

Per serving (1 bun)		% energy
Energy	179 kcal	
Protein	5.3 g	12%
Fat	3.6 g	18%
Carbohydrate	33 g	70%
Fibre	1.1 g	

BREAD

POTATOES

Potatoes are the perfect energy food for athletes. They are high in complex carbohydrate and extremely low in fat. A plain baked potato eaten 30 minutes before your workout will boost blood sugar levels, sustain your energy levels during exercise and delay fatigue. Eaten within two hours after exercise, the carbohydrates will quickly refuel your glycogen stores and speed your recovery.

NUTRITION FACTS

- Almost half of the fibre is found in the skin of potatoes, so once you peel them you lose a good deal of the fibre.
- Potatoes contain lots of potassium and hardly any sodium, which is good for keeping cramps at bay and your blood pressure in check.
- Potatoes are also a great source of vitamin C, thiamin (a B vitamin), magnesium, iron and folic acid.
- New potatoes and freshly dug main crop potatoes contain the most vitamin C, but this steadily falls with storage. Freshly dug potatoes contain 21 mg of vitamin C per 100 g but this drops to 9 mg after three months of storage and 7 mg after nine months. The recommended daily intake of vitamin C is 40 mg.
- You'll lose hefty amounts of vitamin C during peeling, preparation and cooking. A lot of the vitamin C is found just below the skin so cook potatoes in their skins for maximum goodness – bake or boil them in jackets, and leave the skins on when roasting and making chips.
- If you must peel potatoes, do so very thinly and just before cooking. Plunge into fast boiling water and only boil for as long as necessary to make them just soft (do not overcook). Drain and serve straight away.

JUST JACKETS

A jacket potato is one of the simplest, most delicious and most satisfying foods. With crisp skin and floury, tender flesh it makes a great centrepiece for an energy-boosting meal. It is also highly nutritious, providing complex carbohydrates, B vitamins, vitamin C, iron and fibre.

Large potatoes (for a main course allow a 300 g/11 oz potato per person; for a light meal allow a 225 g/8 oz potato per person)
Oil, salt

1 Wash the potatoes and pierce with a fork.

2 For a crispy skin, smear lightly in a very little oil. Rub in a little salt.

3 Bake on the oven shelf at 220°C/425°F/gas mark 7 for 1¼ hours, or until the flesh is very tender.

4 Save time by baking several potatoes at a time. They will keep wrapped in the fridge for up to 3 days.

TWENTY LOW FAT TOPPINGS FOR JACKET POTATOES

1 Baked beans
2 Fromage frais
3 Plain yoghurt, pinch of cayenne pepper
4 Half fat crème fraîche
5 Stir fried vegetables
6 Chicken mixed with fromage frais and paprika
7 Cottage cheese, diced red pepper, chives and sweetcorn
8 Prawns with low calorie salad cream and a dash of tomato sauce
9 Ratatouille (aubergines, courgettes, onions, peppers, tomatoes, garlic)
10 Lentil dahl and plain yoghurt
11 Tuna with plain yoghurt and a dash of chilli sauce
12 Chopped turkey, diced apple and cranberry sauce
13 Grilled mushrooms, fromage frais and freshly ground black pepper
14 Ready-made salsa (mild or hot!)
15 Half a 400 g tin chilli beans in chilli sauce topped with a spoonful of yoghurt
16 1 scrambled egg mixed with a chopped tomato
17 Low fat or fat-free salad dressing
18 Sweetcorn with mixed peppers topped with a spoonful of thick yoghurt
19 Tuna in brine (drained) mixed with 1 tbsp low fat soft cheese or reduced fat mayonnaise
20 Apple sauce

TOMATO AND MUSHROOM TOPPING

You can use 2 tbsp tinned tomatoes instead of fresh tomatoes.

Makes 1 serving
1 tsp olive oil
1 tbsp chopped onion
50 g (2 oz) button mushrooms
1 tomato, chopped
Pinch of dried basil
Freshly ground black pepper

1 Sauté the onion and mushrooms in the oil over a high heat for 3–4 minutes.
2 Add the tomato, herbs and pepper and heat through.

Per serving (including 300 g/11 oz potato)		% energy
Energy	292 kcal	
Protein	8.3 g	11%
Fat	5.2 g	16%
Carbohydrate	56 g	73%
Fibre	5.8 g	

SPICY BEAN TOPPING

Makes 1 serving
2 tbsp salsa (mild or hot)
100 g (4 oz) tinned red kidney beans or pinto beans
1 tbsp Greek yoghurt

Less than 5 minutes to prepare!

1 Combine the salsa and drained beans.
2 Pile onto the potato and top with the Greek yoghurt.

Per serving (including 300 g/11 oz potato)		% energy
Energy	401 kcal	
Protein	16 g	16%
Fat	2.33 g	6%
Carbohydrate	82 g	78%
Fibre	12 g	

SPINACH AND CHEESE TOPPING

Makes 1 serving
100 g (4 oz) fresh or thawed frozen spinach
100 g (4 oz) low fat soft cheese or cottage cheese
Salt and freshly ground black pepper
Ground nutmeg
1 tbsp grated parmesan or mature Cheddar cheese (optional)

Spinach is a rich source of iron

1 Wash the fresh spinach, if applicable. Place the spinach in a saucepan without additional water over a low heat and cook for 2 minutes until wilted.
2 Meanwhile, scoop out the flesh from the jacket potatoes and roughly mash with a fork.
3 Drain any surplus liquid from the spinach. Combine with the potato, soft cheese, salt, pepper and ground nutmeg.
4 Pile the spinach mixture back into the potato shells. Sprinkle with parmesan cheese, if applicable and heat through in the oven or microwave.

Per serving (including 300 g/11 oz potato)		% energy
Energy	379 kcal	
Protein	27 g	29%
Fat	6.5 g	15%
Carbohydrate	56 g	56%
Fibre	0.1 g	

POTATOES

POTATOES

MIGHTY MASH I

This recipe is much lower in fat than the traditional method of using butter and cream.

Low fat version!

Makes I serving
300 g (11 oz) potato, peeled
100 ml (4 fl oz) skimmed milk
Salt and freshly ground
black pepper
Dash of tabasco sauce

1 Cut the potato into rough pieces and cook in a little fast boiling water for 10–15 minutes, or until tender. Drain.
2 Mash together the potato, most of the milk and seasonings. Add a little extra milk for a softer consistency.

Per serving		% energy
Energy	266 kcal	
Protein	10 g	16%
Fat	0.7 g	3%
Carbohydrate	58 g	81%
Fibre	3.9 g	

MIGHTY MASH II

The combination of potato with other root vegetables not only tastes delicious but boosts the vitamin content too.

Makes I serving
175 g (6 oz) potato, peeled
175 g (6 oz) swede, peeled
1 carrot/1 parsnip (optional)
4 tbsp skimmed milk
Salt and freshly ground
black pepper
Dash of tabasco

1 Cut the potato and swede into rough pieces and cook in a little fast boiling water for 10 minutes, or until soft. Drain.
2 Mash together the potato, swede (and carrot or parsnip, if applicable), milk and seasonings. Add a little extra milk for a softer consistency.

Per serving		% energy
Energy	193 kcal	
Protein	6.9 g	14%
Fat	0.9 g	4%
Carbohydrate	42 g	82%
Fibre	5.6 g	

CHUNKY OVEN CHIPS

These low fat chips are healthy and deli-cious; they retain all their vitamin C as no peeling is required.

Makes I serving

I large potato, scrubbed
I tsp sunflower or olive oil
Salt/garlic powder/parmesan cheese/chilli powder (all optional)

I Cut the potato lengthways, then cut each half into 6 wedges.
2 Place in a baking tin and baste in the oil until each piece is coated.
3 Bake at 200°C/400°F/gas mark 6 for 20–25 minutes until the potatoes are soft inside and golden brown on the outside.
4 Sprinkle on any one of the optional ingredients 5 minutes before the end of cooking.

Per serving		% energy
Energy	205 kcal	
Protein	4.7 g	9%
Fat	4.6 g	20%
Carbohydrate	39 g	71%
Fibre	2.9 g	

ATHLETE'S BUBBLE AND SQUEAK

Bursting with flavour and goodness, this recipe is a terrific way to use up any left-over vegetables. It is also an ideal method of disguising green vegetables for those who are not keen on them!

Makes I serving

225 g (8 oz) potato
225 g (8 oz) green leafy vegetables, e.g. cabbage, spinach, Brussels sprouts, spring greens
3–4 tbsp skimmed milk
Salt and freshly ground black pepper
Chopped parsley

I Peel and chop the potatoes and other vegetables.
2 Boil in a little fast boiling water for 10–15 minutes, or until tender. Drain, reserving the liquid for soups, stock, etc.
3 Mash with the milk and seasoning.
4 Spoon into a small ovenproof dish, level the surface and grill until the top is crispy (optional).

Per serving		% energy
Energy	249 kcal	
Protein	11 g	18%
Fat	1.6 g	6%
Carbohydrate	50 g	76%
Fibre	9.9 g	

POTATOES

POTATO GRIDDLE SCONES

Eat these as an accompaniment to a main meal or as a savoury snack. Delicious on their own or spread with a little butter, fromage frais or jam. They are rich in complex carbohydrate.

Makes 8 scones

450 g (1lb) potatoes, boiled
4 tbsp skimmed milk
100 g (4 oz) plain white flour
Salt and freshly ground
black pepper

1 Mash the potatoes with the milk until very smooth.
2 Add the flour, salt and black pepper and mix together with your hands until it forms a soft dough.
3 Roll out and cut into 8 circles using a scone cutter of approximately 7½ cm (3 in) diameter.
4 Heat a non-stick frying pan or griddle and cook the scones until lightly browned on both sides.

Per serving (1 scone)		% energy
Energy	98 kcal	
Protein	2.9 g	12%
Fat	0.3 g	5%
Carbohydrate	22 g	85%
Fibre	1.2 g	

POTATO TACOS

Add a green vegetable such as broccoli or green cabbage to give a vitamin C boost to the meal.

Makes 1 serving

1 large (275 g/10 oz) baking potato
Half a tin (210 g) red kidney or pinto beans
2 tbsp mild taco sauce (ready-made)
25 g (1 oz) grated Cheddar cheese
2 tbsp plain low fat yoghurt
Shredded iceberg lettuce
Finely chopped fresh tomato
1 canned chilli, sliced (optional)

1 Scrub the potato and prick with a fork. Smear with a little oil and salt – this gives a crispy jacket. Bake in a hot oven (200°C/400°F/gas mark 6) for 1 hour.
2 Drain the beans and heat in a pan with the taco sauce.
3 Split the cooked potato. Spoon on the beans and sauce.
4 Top with the grated cheese and yoghurt. Scatter with the lettuce, tomato and chilli (if you can take the heat!).

Per serving		% energy
Energy	527 kcal	
Protein	25 g	19%
Fat	11 g	18%
Carbohydrate	87 g	63%
Fibre	14 g	

PERFECT POTATO PIE

Prepare this dish in advance. It can cook while you go out for a run or have a bath – don't worry if you leave it for longer than 60 minutes as the cooking time isn't too important.

Makes 4 servings

1 kg (2.2 lb) potatoes
600 ml (1 pint) skimmed milk
50 g (2 oz) grated cheese
1 onion, thinly sliced
2 eggs
Salt and freshly ground
black pepper
Sliced leeks/broccoli florets/sliced
tomatoes (all optional)

1 Peel and slice the potatoes. Arrange layers of potato, cheese and onion (and any optional vegetables) in a shallow baking dish, finishing with the cheese.

2 Beat the eggs with the milk, season and pour over the potatoes.

3 Cover with foil and bake at 200°C/400°F/gas mark 6 for 45–60 minutes until the potatoes are tender and the top golden brown.

Per serving		% energy
Energy	348 kcal	
Protein	18 g	21%
Fat	9.1 g	23%
Carbohydrate	52 g	56%
Fibre	3.5 g	

GARLIC ROAST POTATOES

The garlic contains powerful anti-cancer and heart protective compounds.

Makes 1 serving

1 large potato (approx. 300 g)
1 tsp olive oil
1 garlic clove, crushed

1 Cut the potato into chunks (no need to peel).

2 Place the oil and crushed garlic in a roasting tin and baste the potato chunks so they are evenly coated with oil.

3 Bake in the oven at 200°C/400°F/gas mark 6 for 45 minutes or until golden brown.

Per serving		% energy
Energy	261 kcal	
Protein	6.3 g	10%
Fat	4.6 g	16%
Carbohydrate	52 g	74%
Fibre	3.9 g	

POTATOES

POTATO KUGEL

A vegetable kugel is a basic Jewish dish; a shallow casserole pudding that is held together with beaten egg, has a crispy top and is cut into squares. This adaptation of the classic potato kugel is ideal for increasing your carbohydrate intake.

Makes 4 servings

4 large potatoes (approx. 225 g/ 8 oz each)
2 onions, chopped
1 tbsp oil
Salt and freshly ground black pepper
4 eggs
300 ml (½ pint) fromage frais or plain yoghurt
50 g (2 oz) fresh breadcrumbs
225 g (8 oz) mushrooms/ courgettes/grated carrots (all optional)

1 Scrub and coarsely grate the potatoes in a bowl.

2 Sauté the onion in the oil over a moderate heat for 4–5 minutes together with any of the optional ingredients. Add to the grated potato.

3 Add the seasoning, eggs, fromage frais and breadcrumbs. Combine well.

4 Spread evenly into an oiled 9 × 13 in baking tin. Dust the top with paprika.

5 Bake at 190°C/375°F/gas mark 5 for 1 hour or until crisp on the top. Cut into squares and serve.

Per serving		% energy
Energy	389 kcal	
Protein	20 g	21%
Fat	10 g	23%
Carbohydrate	58 g	56%
Fibre	3.7 g	

COD AND POTATO PIE

Serve this with lightly cooked broccoli or green cabbage to add extra vitamins.

Makes 4 servings

550 g (1¼ lb) potatoes, peeled
600 ml (1 pint) skimmed milk
2 large leeks, thinly sliced
550 g (1¼ lb) cod fillets
1 bay leaf
2 heaped tbsp plain flour
Salt and freshly ground black pepper
Dijon mustard
50 g (2 oz) mature Cheddar cheese, grated

1 Chop and cook the potatoes in a little fast-boiling water for 10–15 minutes, or until soft. Drain and mash with a little of the milk.

2 Meanwhile, place the cod and leeks in a saucepan with the remaining milk and bay leaf. Bring to the boil and simmer for 5 minutes.

3 Strain the milk into a jug. Roughly flake the fish.

4 Stir the flour into the milk, return to the pan and bring to the boil, stirring until the sauce has thickened. Season with salt, pepper and Dijon mustard.

5 Combine the sauce with the leeks and fish. Place in a baking dish.

6 Cover evenly with the mashed potatoes and scatter the cheese on top.

7 Bake at 190°C/375°F/gas mark 5 for 20 minutes or until the top is golden brown.

Per serving		% energy
Energy	367 kcal	
Protein	38 g	42%
Fat	6.9 g	3%
Carbohydrate	40 g	41%
Fibre	3 g	

VEGETABLE CRUMBLE

A perfect warming winter dish that makes a nutritionally complete meal. The seeds and nuts in the topping are excellent sources of essential fatty acids.

Makes 4 servings

Filling:
  1 kg (2.2 lb) mixed root
  vegetables, e.g. potato, carrot,
  turnip, parsnip, swede
  25 g (1 oz) butter or margarine
  25 g (1 oz) flour
  300 ml (½ pint) skimmed or semi-
  skimmed milk
  ½ tsp Marmite
  Salt and freshly ground
  black pepper
  Fresh parsley
Crumble:
  75 g (3 oz) wholemeal flour
  25 g (1 oz) oats
  25 g (1 oz) butter or margarine
  1 tbsp sunflower seeds/flaked
  almonds/peanuts (all optional)

1 Slice the vegetables thickly and cook in boiling water for 15 minutes, or until just tender. Drain, reserving 250 ml (8 fl oz) cooking liquid.

2 Melt the butter or margarine in a pan, stir in the flour and cook for 1–2 minutes. Slowly add the milk and reserved water, stirring continuously.

3 Add the Marmite, salt, pepper and parsley to taste.

4 Spoon the vegetables and sauce into a large casserole dish.

5 To make the crumble, mix the oats and flour together. Rub in the butter or margarine then stir in the remaining ingredients.

6 Sprinkle over the vegetables and bake at 200°C/400°F/gas mark 6 for 30 minutes.

Per serving		% energy
Energy	340 kcal	
Protein	9.6 g	11%
Fat	12.4 g	33%
Carbohydrate	51 g	56%
Fibre	8.6 g	

POTATOES

VEGETABLE GRATIN WITH POTATOES

A good way of serving vegetables to those who do not like them plain. The gratin topping can be used with any variety of vegetables.

Makes 4 servings

1 cauliflower, cut into florets
450 g (1 lb) broccoli, cut into florets
450 ml (¾ pint) skimmed milk
2 tbsp cornflour
1 tsp mustard
50 g (2 oz) mature Cheddar cheese
900 g (2 lb) potatoes
1 tbsp sesame seeds/walnuts (optional)

1 Cook the cauliflower and broccoli in boiling water for 5 minutes. Drain and reserve the liquid.
2 Blend the cornflour with a little of the milk. Gradually add the remaining milk and transfer into a saucepan.
3 Heat, stirring constantly, until the sauce thickens. Add the mustard, three quarters of the cheese and some of the reserved cooking liquid to give a coating consistency.
4 Arrange the vegetables in a baking dish, pour over the sauce and sprinkle with the remaining cheese and optional seeds or nuts.
5 Place under a hot grill until golden brown.
6 Serve with cooked potatoes.

Per serving		% energy
Energy	368 kcal	
Protein	20 g	22%
Fat	7.9 g	19%
Carbohydrate	57 g	59%
Fibre	8.7 g	

POTATO AND VEGETABLE CURRY

This ultra-quick curry can be made with any combination of vegetables.

Makes 4 servings

675 g (1½ lb) potatoes
1 onion, chopped
1 tbsp olive oil
450 g (1 lb) vegetables, e.g. peas, mushrooms, sweetcorn, mange tout, green beans
1 tbsp curry powder
1 tin (400 g) chopped tomatoes

1 Cut the potatoes into small chunks. Sauté the potatoes and onion in the oil in a large frying pan for 4–5 minutes.
2 Add the remaining ingredients, stir, bring to the boil and simmer for 15 minutes, or until the potatoes and vegetables are tender.

Per serving		% energy
Energy	240 kcal	
Protein	9 g	15%
Fat	4.5 g	17%
Carbohydrate	43 g	68%
Fibre	6.5 g	

AUBERGINE AND POTATO CURRY

Cooking the aubergine over a high heat prevents it absorbing lots of oil. Aubergines are good sources of folic acid and potassium.

Makes 4 servings

1 tbsp butter or olive oil
2 onions, chopped
1 aubergine, cut into cubes
1 tbsp curry powder
8 new potatoes, cut into halves
1 tbsp tomato purée
50 ml (2 fl oz) water
175 g (6 oz) frozen peas

1 Heat the butter or oil in a large pan and cook the onions and aubergine over a high heat until soft, about 6–8 minutes.
2 Add the curry powder and potatoes and cook for 1 minute.
3 Add the water, tomato purée and peas and cook until the potatoes are tender and the curry has thickened.
4 Serve with plain yoghurt and chapattis or naan bread.

Per serving		% energy
Energy	141 kcal	
Protein	5.3 g	15%
Fat	3.7 g	24%
Carbohydrate	23 g	61%
Fibre	5 g	

POTATO SALAD

This is an excellent portable snack or lunch. Accompany with a protein food such as cooked chicken drumsticks, boiled eggs or cottage cheese, and some vegetable crudités for a nutritionally complete meal on the run.

Makes 1 serving

225 g (8 oz) new or old potatoes, cut into small chunks (no need to peel)
1 tbsp each of fresh chopped mint and parsley (or use 1 tsp dried)
1 tbsp plain yoghurt
1 tbsp reduced calorie salad cream or mayonnaise
Freshly ground black pepper
Chopped spring onions/onions/cucumber/peppers (all optional)

1 Boil the potatoes in a little fast-boiling water for 5–7 minutes until just tender. Drain.
2 Combine the remaining ingredients together. Toss in the cooled potatoes and any of the optional ingredients.

Per serving		% energy
Energy	211 kcal	
Protein	5.4 g	10%
Fat	4.4 g	19%
Carbohydrate	40 g	71%
Fibre	2.8 g	

POTATOES

POTATOES

POTATO BAKE WITH TOMATOES

An excellent source of complex carbohy-drates, vitamin C and fibre. The olive oil not only adds a delicious flavour but also valuable monounsaturates.

Makes 4 servings

900 g (2 lb) potatoes
4 large tomatoes, sliced
Handful of fresh herbs, e.g. parsley, rosemary, basil
Salt and freshly ground
black pepper
2 tbsp olive oil
One small glass of white wine (or water)
4 tbsp breadcrumbs (optional)

1 Boil the potatoes in their skins for 5 minutes. Cool then slice thickly.

2 Layer the potatoes and tomatoes in a baking dish. Sprinkle salt, black pepper and herbs between the layers.

3 Pour the olive oil and wine over the vegetables. Sprinkle with the breadcrumbs, if applicable.

4 Bake at 180°C/350°F/gas mark 4 for 20 minutes or until the potatoes are soft. Alternatively, microwave for 8 minutes.

Per serving		% energy
Energy	255 kcal	
Protein	5.5 g	9%
Fat	6.3 g	22%
Carbohydrate	42 g	61%
Fibre	4 g	

PIE CRUSTS AND PASTRY SUBSTITUTES

Traditional pastry is loaded with fat and has no place in an athlete's daily diet. Here are some ideas for low fat pie crusts which you can substitute for pastry when making pies and quiches, and safely include in your sports diet. Many do not require the traditional rolling out – you simply pat them into the baking tin with a spoon, fork or your fingers. Fill and bake in the usual way.

Fillings – Ham and Mushroom Sauce (p. 157), Quick Tuna and Sweetcorn Sauce (p. 155) or Chicken and Mushroom Sauce (p. 157)

POTATO PASTRY

450 g (1 lb) potatoes, peeled and roughly chopped
100 g (4 oz) self raising flour
½ tsp baking powder
1 egg
Salt and freshly ground black pepper

1 Boil the potatoes for 10–15 minutes until just tender. Drain and mash. Cool slightly.

2 Mix the potato with the flour, baking powder, seasoning and enough egg to form a soft dough. Allow to cool completely.

3 Roll out or press into the baking tin. Bake at 190°C/375°F/gas mark 5 for 30 minutes.

Per ¼ recipe		% energy
Energy	209 kcal	
Protein	7 g	13%
Fat	2.2 g	10%
Carbohydrate	43 g	77%
Fibre	2.4 g	

MASHED POTATO PIE CRUST

Use any of the fillings suggested on page 187.

450 g (1 lb) potatoes
2 tbsp butter or margarine
Salt and freshly ground
black pepper
1 small onion, finely chopped

1 Scrub the potatoes, cut into chunks and boil them until just soft. Drain and mash.

2 Combine with the butter, seasoning and onion.

3 Press into the baking tin using a spoon or spatula. Bake at 190°C/375°F/gas mark 5 for 45 minutes.

Per ¼ recipe		% energy
Energy	125 kcal	
Protein	2.5 g	8%
Fat	4.3 g	31%
Carbohydrate	20 g	61%
Fibre	1.6 g	

CRUNCHY PIE CRUST

Fill this pie crust with thinly sliced tomatoes, sprinkled with a little olive oil, freshly ground black pepper and fresh basil leaves. Alternatively use a traditional quiche filling.

50 g (2 oz) fresh wholemeal breadcrumbs
25 g (1 oz) wholemeal flour
25 g (1 oz) wheatgerm
25 g (1 oz) oats
Pinch of salt and dried basil
40 g (1½ oz) melted butter/low fat spread

1 Mix together all the dry ingredients.

2 Drizzle in the melted butter and mix with a fork until the mixture is

evenly coated. Add a little water if necessary.

3 Press into the baking tin. Bake at 180°C/350°F/gas mark 4 for 10 minutes.

Per ¼ recipe		% energy
Energy	193 kcal	
Protein	5 g	10%
Fat	9.6 g	45%
Carbohydrate	23 g	45%
Fibre	1.3 g	

VEGETABLE PIE CRUST

This tasty crust goes well with creamy fillings. Try Cheese Sauce (p. 156) combined with ham or boiled quartered eggs.

1 large parsnip, grated
2 carrots, grated
100 g (4 oz) swede, grated
½ tsp salt
2 tbsp melted butter or margarine
40 g (1½ oz) wholemeal flour

1 Combine all of the ingredients and mix well.

2 Press into a lightly-oiled baking tin and form a pie crust with your fingers. Bake at 190°C/375°F/gas mark 5 for 40 minutes.

Per ¼ recipe		% energy
Energy	112 kcal	
Protein	2.4 g	9%
Fat	4.9 g	39%
Carbohydrate	16 g	52%
Fibre	4.1 g	

BREAKFAST

It's been proven that a high carbohydrate, low fat breakfast improves your mood, concentration and your physical and mental performance. Breakfast-eaters are leaner than those who skip this important meal and have higher intakes of most vitamins and minerals. If you cannot face breakfast very early in the day, aim to eat within two hours of waking.

HOW POPULAR BREAKFASTS COMPARE	
COOKED BREAKFAST	**CONTINENTAL BREAKFAST**
2 rashers fried streaky bacon 2 fried eggs 1 grilled tomato 2 slices white toast with butter 600 kcal; 44 g fat; 8.5 g sugars; 3 g fibre	2 croissants 20 g butter 20 g jam 612 kcal; 37 g fat; 29 g sugars; 1.6 g fibre
TOAST AND MARMALADE	**BREAKFAST CEREAL**
2 slices white toast 20 g butter 20 g marmalade 395 kcal; 17 g fat; 30 g sugars; 1.1 g fibre	1 bowl (50 g) bran flakes 125 ml semi-skimmed milk 218 kcal; 3 g fat; 18 g sugars; 6.5 g fibre 2 Weetabix 125 ml semi-skimmed milk 180 kcal; 3 g fat; 8 g sugars; 5 g fibre

TOP TIPS FOR A HEALTHY BREAKFAST

- Always include at least one portion of fruit with your breakfast, e.g. 1 banana, 1 apple, 1 orange, 100 g (4 oz) strawberries.
- Include at least one high carbohydrate food, e.g. breakfast cereal, porridge oats, toast, bread, English muffins, bagels, pancakes, waffles.
- If you aren't keen on high fibre cereals, mix your favourite low fibre cereal with a cereal providing at least 7 g fibre/100 g.
- Use semi-skimmed milk or skimmed milk instead of full fat milk.
- Avoid fried foods, e.g. bacon, sausages and high fat foods, e.g. croissants, pastries.
- Add dried fruit, e.g. raisins, dates, prunes, instead of sugar to sweeten your cereal. You'll also get extra fibre and vitamins.

OATMAL SCOTTIES

Oatmeal provides slow-releasing energy – a perfect start to an active day. It's also rich in soluble fibre, iron and B vitamins.

Makes 12 small pancakes

175 g (6 oz) fine oatmeal
100 g (4 oz) plain wholemeal flour
2 tsp baking powder
350 ml (12 fl oz) buttermilk or half yoghurt/half skimmed milk
2 egg whites

1 Combine the oatmeal, flour and baking powder in a bowl or liquidiser.

2 Whisk together the buttermilk and egg whites. Add to the flour and blend until smooth.

3 If you have time, let the batter stand for about 10 minutes.

4 Heat a large non-stick frying pan or cast-iron griddle and smear with a little oil or oil spray.

5 Drop spoonfuls of the batter into the pan to make small pancakes 10–12 cm (4–5 in) diameter. You

should be able to cook 3–4 pancakes at once.

6 Cook for approximately 2 minutes on a high heat until the pancakes are golden brown underneath. Turn over and cook for 1 more minute.

7 Keep warm on a plate while you make the other pancakes.

Topping variations

- Scrambled eggs mixed with chopped tomatoes.
- Mashed or sliced bananas.
- Apricot fruit spread and cottage cheese.
- Sautéed mushrooms mixed with half fat crème fraîche.

Per serving (1 pancake)		% energy
Energy	103 kcal	
Protein	4.6 g	18%
Fat	1.6 g	14%
Carbohydrate	19 g	68%
Fibre	1.9 g	

BREAKFAST BAGELS

Bagels are low in fat and high in carbo-hydrate – to help keep you going until lunch! There are lots of different kinds of bagel to choose from – raisin and cinnamon, onion, sesame, plain, blueberry – to name but a few. Here are some ideas for healthy toppings:

- Honey
- Cottage cheese with pineapple
- Peanut butter
- Thinly sliced salmon and cucumber
- Sliced banana and low fat soft cheese
- Marmite and sliced cheese
- Fruit conserve or fruit spread

BREAKFAST MUFFINS

These take only a few minutes to make and are excellent for a weekend breakfast treat. See also other muffin recipes on pages 225–8.

Makes 12 muffins

100 g (4 oz) white self raising flour
100 g (4 oz) wholemeal self raising flour
1 tbsp (15 ml) oil
40 g (1½ oz) soft brown sugar
1 egg
150 ml (5 fl oz) skimmed milk
50 g (2 oz) dried fruit

1 Preheat the oven to 220°C/425°F/gas mark 7.
2 Mix the flours together in a bowl.
3 Add the oil, sugar, egg and milk. Mix well.
4 Stir in the dried fruit.
5 Spoon into a non-stick muffin tray and bake for approximately 15 minutes until golden brown.

Per serving (1 muffin)		% energy
Energy	109 kcal	
Protein	3 g	11%
Fat	1.8 g	15%
Carbohydrate	22 g	74%
Fibre	1.4 g	

DRIED FRUIT MUESLI

Makes 10 servings

100 g (4 oz) dried fruit
350 g (12 oz) porridge oats
150 g (5 oz) wheat flakes or bran flakes
65 g (2½ oz) wheatgerm
50 g (2 oz) each of raisins, dates and figs

1 Chop the dried fruit.
2 Put all the ingredients in a bowl and mix well.
3 Store in an airtight container.
4 Serve with low fat milk or low fat milk mixed with bioyoghurt.

Variations

- Substitute dried fruit (e.g. apples, pears, mango, apricot, pineapple) for the dried fruit mixture.

Per serving		% energy
Energy	284 kcal	
Protein	8.8 g	12%
Fat	4.2 g	13%
Carbohydrate	56 g	75%
Fibre	7.2 g	

BREAKFAST

BREAKFAST PANCAKES

These pancakes are made with wholemeal flour to boost the vitamin and fibre content. You can use fine oatmeal instead of wholemeal flour for a nuttier flavour.

Makes 6 pancakes

Batter:
  65 g (2½ oz) plain white flour
  65 g (2½ oz) plain wholemeal flour
  1 egg
  300 ml (½ pint) skimmed milk
  (A little vegetable oil or oil spray for frying)
Filling:
  1 orange, peeled and cut into segments
  1 ruby grapefruit, peeled and cut into segments
  1 banana, peeled and sliced
  1–2 tbsp clear honey

1 Place all the batter ingredients in a liquidiser and blend until smooth. Alternatively mix the flours in a bowl. Make a well in the centre. Beat the egg and milk and gradually add to the flour, beating to make a smooth batter.

2 Place a non-stick frying pan over a high heat. Spray with oil spray or add a few drops of oil.

3 Pour in enough batter to coat the pan thinly and cook for 1–2 minutes until golden brown on the underside.

4 Turn the pancake and cook the other side for 30–60 seconds.

5 Turn out onto a plate, cover and keep warm while you make the other pancakes.

6 To make the fillings, combine the chopped fruit with the honey.

7 Divide the fruit between the pancakes and fold them in half. Serve topped with low fat yoghurt.

Filling variations

• 1 banana mixed with 1 sliced peach and 1 tbsp honey.

• 8 fresh chopped apricots mixed with a 100 g (4 oz) carton of very low fat apricot yoghurt.

• 100 g (4 oz) sliced strawberries mixed with 100 g (4 oz) very low fat fromage frais.

• 100 g (4 oz) summer fruit.

Per serving (1 pancake)		% energy
Energy	155 kcal	
Protein	6.2 g	16%
Fat	1.6 g	10%
Carbohydrate	31 g	74%
Fibre	2.4 g	

BANANA WAFFLES

Waffles are a great weekend treat when you have more time. Make a larger quantity and freeze the remainder for weekday snacks.

Makes 4 large waffles

225 ml (8 fl oz) semi-skimmed milk
1 egg
2 tsp oil
75 g (3 oz) self raising white or wholemeal flour
1 tsp sugar
Pinch of cinnamon
2 bananas
Equipment: waffle iron

1 Beat together the milk, egg and oil.

2 Mix together the flour, sugar and cinnamon.

3 Beat the liquid mixture into the flour mixture until smooth. Alternatively blend in a liquidiser.

4 Heat the waffle iron and spray or lightly smear with oil.

5 Spoon one quarter of the mixture into each waffle compartment.

Cook for approximately 2 minutes until golden and beginning to separate from the waffle iron. Repeat with the remainder of the mixture.

6 Top the waffles with sliced bananas.

Topping variations

- Maple syrup or honey and sliced strawberries.
- Cottage cheese mixed with chopped apricots.
- Blueberry fruit spread.

Per serving (1 waffle)		% energy
Energy	191 kcal	
Protein	6.5 g	14%
Fat	5 g	23%
Carbohydrate	32 g	63%
Fibre	1.2 g	

APPLE SAUCE MUFFINS

You can use sliced bananas instead of the apple sauce.

1 wholemeal English muffin
2 tbsp low fat soft cheese or ricotta cheese
2 tbsp unsweetened apple sauce (bought or home-made)
Cinnamon

1 Split the muffin in half and toast lightly under a hot grill.

2 Spread the muffin halves with the cheese and apple sauce.

3 Sprinkle with cinnamon and pop under the grill to heat through.

Per serving		% energy
Energy	276 kcal	
Protein	11 g	16%
Fat	8.8 g	28%
Carbohydrate	41 g	56%
Fibre	2.6 g	

BASIC GRANOLA

Shop-bought versions use palm oil (a highly saturated fat) or hydrogenated fat. This recipe uses sunflower oil.

Healthier than shop-bought version

Makes 10 servings

450 g (1 lb) oats
50 g (2 oz) brown sugar or honey
1 tsp cinnamon (optional)
3 tbsp sunflower oil
4 tbsp water
1 tsp vanilla
100 g (4 oz) bran flakes or wheat flakes
100 g (4 oz) raisins, sultanas, chopped dates, chopped figs or dried apricots/100 g (4 oz) dried apple/75 g (3 oz) chopped toasted hazelnuts or flaked toasted almonds/50 g (2 oz) toasted sunflower seeds (all optional)

1 Combine the oats, sugar (or honey), cinnamon, oil, water and vanilla in a large bowl.

2 Spread thinly over two baking trays.

3 Bake for 30–35 minutes at 150°C/300°F/gas mark 2, stirring halfway through to ensure an even toasting.

4 Allow to cool, then stir in the bran or wheat flakes. Stir in the optional ingredients and store in an airtight container.

Per serving		% energy
Energy	274 kcal	
Protein	6.9 g	10%
Fat	7.5 g	25%
Carbohydrate	48 g	65%
Fibre	4.7 g	

BREAKFAST

POWER PORRIDGE

Oats provide slow-releasing energy, soluble fibre, iron and B vitamins.

Makes 1 large serving

50 g (2 oz) porridge oats
350 ml (12 fl oz) skimmed milk
25 g (1 oz) raisins, dates or figs
1 banana, sliced
2 tsp honey or maple syrup

1 Mix the oats and milk together. Cook in a microwave for approximately 4 minutes, stirring halfway through, or in a saucepan for approximately 5 minutes, stirring continuously.

2 Add the raisins, banana and extra milk if desired.

3 Spoon the honey or maple syrup over the top.

BREAKFAST BARS

These tasty bars will keep well in an air-tight container for up to 5 days.

For breakfast on the move!

Makes 12 bars

100 g (4 oz) dried apricots, chopped
100 g (4 oz) dates, chopped
1 egg
1 tbsp oil
100 ml (4 fl oz) plain yoghurt
50 g (2 oz) sugar
50 g (2 oz) self raising wholemeal flour
4 Weetabix, crumbled

1 Combine the apricots, dates, egg, oil and yoghurt in a bowl. Mix well.

2 Stir in the sugar, flour and Weetabix. Add a little milk if the mixture is too stiff.

3 Spoon into a lightly-oiled non-stick 8 in square baking dish.

4 Bake at 190°C/375°F/gas mark 5 for 20–25 minutes.

5 Cool and cut into bars.

Per serving		% energy
Energy	562 kcal	
Protein	21 g	15%
Fat	6 g	10%
Carbohydrate	113 g	75%
Fibre	5.7 g	

Per serving (1 bar)		% energy
Energy	129 kcal	
Protein	3.2 g	10%
Fat	1.9 g	13%
Carbohydrate	26 g	77%
Fibre	2 g	

BAKED FRENCH TOAST

You can use any type of bread for this recipe, such as raisin bread, wholemeal bread or French bread.

Makes 2 servings

4 thick slices white bread
3 eggs
300 ml (½ pint) skimmed milk
½ tsp cinnamon

1 Spray a 9 in square baking tray with oil spray or lightly smear with oil.
2 Cut the bread slices in half diagonally and arrange them in layers on the tray.

3 Whisk together the eggs, milk and cinnamon. Pour over the bread.
4 Bake for 25–30 minutes at 180°C/350°F/gas mark 4. (This recipe may be made the night before and refrigerated until the morning.) Serve with apple sauce or chopped fresh fruit.

Per serving		% energy
Energy	352 kcal	
Protein	23 g	26%
Fat	11 g	28%
Carbohydrate	43 g	46%
Fibre	1.1 g	

CEREAL TOPPINGS

Top ready-made cereals with any of the following to add extra carbohydrate, fibre, vitamins and minerals.

- Dried fruit, e.g. raisins, pineapple, apple, dates, figs
- Sliced bananas
- Fresh fruit, e.g. strawberries, raspberries, peaches, oranges
- Plain or fruit yoghurt
- Nuts, sunflower or pumpkin seeds

FIVE-MINUTE MEALS AND LUNCH ON THE GO

The following recipes can all be assembled in a few minutes or less. They are ideal for nutritious snacks, lunch on the go, or even a quick supper when you haven't got time to cook.

QUICK TACOS

You can use tinned refried beans instead of the salsa and pinto beans.

Makes 2 tacos

2 tbsp chunky Mexican salsa
Half a tin (210 g) pinto or red kidney beans
2 taco shells
Diced tomato, shredded lettuce, beansprouts
2 tbsp grated cheese

1 Combine the salsa and beans in a pan and heat through.
2 Meanwhile heat the tacos in a hot oven for a few minutes.
3 Spoon the salsa into the taco shells and serve topped with the tomatoes, lettuce, beansprouts and cheese.

Per serving		% energy
Energy	386 kcal	
Protein	19 g	20%
Fat	8.5 g	20%
Carbohydrate	62 g	60%
Fibre	11.5 g	

BAGEL MELT

I bagel
2 thin slices (40 g/1½ oz) Cheddar
cheese

Makes I serving

1 Split the bagel in half.
2 Lay the cheese slices on the cut
   sides and toast under a hot grill until
   melted.
3 Sandwich the two halves back
   together.
4 Alternatively, place the cheese
   between the bagel halves and
   microwave until melted.

Variations

• Spread the split bagel with peanut
  butter before adding the cheese.
• Place six slices of beef tomatoes
  over the cheese before toasting.
• Scatter thin slices of onion or
  shallot over the cheese before
  toasting.
• Add chopped lettuce, cucumber and
  tomato to the melted cheese before
  sandwiching together.

Per serving		% energy
Energy	331 kcal	
Protein	14 g	17%
Fat	12 g	33%
Carbohydrate	44 g	50%
Fibre	1.3 g	

BANANA HOT DOG

I long roll, preferably wholemeal,
e.g. Hoagie
Butter/low fat spread
I banana

Makes I serving

To balance
the meal add a
simple salad and
a yoghurt for
dessert

1 Split the roll in half
   and spread thinly
   with the butter or
   low fat spread.
2 Place a whole banana inside.
3 Eat cold or microwave for 10–20
   seconds to warm through.

Per serving		% energy
Energy	339 kcal	
Protein	9.4 g	11%
Fat	6.8 g	18%
Carbohydrate	64 g	71%
Fibre	3.9 g	

TURKEY POCKETS

*You can use chicken instead of turkey if
not available.*

Makes I serving

I large or 2 mini wholemeal pittas
I tbsp (15 ml) low fat salad
dressing
2 slices (50 g/2 oz) turkey breast
Salad leaves

1 Toast then split the pittas.
2 Spread with salad dressing and layer
   turkey and salad leaves.

Per serving		% energy
Energy	290 kcal	
Protein	21 g	29%
Fat	4.1 g	13%
Carbohydrate	45 g	58%
Fibre	3.9 g	

IT'S A WRAP!

Wraps are great alternative to sandwiches. Here are some ideas for healthy fillings:

- Chopped cooked chicken combined with soft cheese and sliced tomato
- Chopped cooked turkey mixed with tzatziki and mango chutney
- Hummus, sliced tomato and shredded lettuce
- Ready-prepared chicken tikka with salad leaves
- Tinned refried beans, grated cheese and shredded lettuce

See pages 70–1 for more ideas.

GREEK FILLED PITTA

Wholemeal pitta bread will give you three times more fibre as well as more B vitamins and iron, compared with white.

   1 large pitta
   1 tbsp (15 ml) hummus (reduced fat)
   25 g (1 oz) crumbled feta cheese
   Baby spinach leaves

1 Toast and split the pitta.
2 Spread with the hummus and fill with the feta cheese and baby spinach.

Per serving		% energy
Energy	332 kcal	
Protein	15 g	18%
Fat	10 g	28%
Carbohydrate	48 g	54%
Fibre	5.9 g	

CURRIED CHICKEN BAGUETTE

Make this into a panini by toasting the assembled baguette in a mini grill machine.

   1 small baguette (approx. 6–8 in)
   1 tbsp (15 ml) low fat salad dressing or mayonnaise
   50 g (2 oz) chopped cooked chicken
   ¼ tsp curry powder
   1 stick of celery, finely chopped

1 Split the baguette.
2 Combine the dressing, chicken, curry powder and celery. Fill the baguette.

Per serving		% energy
Energy	399 kcal	
Protein	28 g	28%
Fat	8.3 g	18%
Carbohydrate	57 g	54%
Fibre	1.8 g	

QUESADILLA

2 corn tortillas
40 g (1½ oz) Edam, Gouda or
reduced fat Cheddar cheese,
grated or sliced
1 tbsp ready-made tomato salsa or
mild taco sauce

1 Place half the cheese and salsa on
each tortilla.

2 Roll up and heat in a microwave/
under the grill until the cheese is
melted.

Variations

• Add chopped spring onions to the
filling.

• Add a few slices of avocado to the
filling.

• Add a handful of shredded white
cabbage to the filling.

• Substitute 1 tbsp (15 ml) of fromage
frais for the tomato salsa.

Per serving		% energy
Energy	308 kcal	
Protein	15 g	19%
Fat	11 g	31%
Carbohydrate	40 g	50%
Fibre	1.6 g	

MUFFIN PIZZA

1 wholemeal English muffin
1 tbsp passata (smooth sieved
tomatoes) or pasta sauce
25 g (1 oz) reduced fat mozzarella
or Edam, sliced
Pinch of dried basil or mixed herbs

1 Split and toast the muffin. Spread
passata or sauce over each cut side.

2 Place the cheese on top and sprinkle
with the herbs.

3 Pop under a hot grill until the
cheese has melted.

Add any available vegetables to the
pizza topping, such as thinly sliced
red, green or yellow peppers, sliced
onions and mushrooms.

Per serving		% energy
Energy	264 kcal	
Protein	16 g	24%
Fat	7.6 g	26%
Carbohydrate	36 g	50%
Fibre	1.5 g	

BEAN AND CORN QUESADILLAS

*The ultimate healthy grilled cheese
sandwiches.*

Makes 4 quesadillas

1 tin (420 g) red kidney or pinto
beans, drained
4 tbsp salsa
8 flour tortillas
100 g (4 oz) Cheddar cheese, grated
1 tbsp vegetable oil

1 Mash the beans roughly with the
salsa until well combined.

2 Divide the filling between four
tortillas. Spread all over the surface,
leaving a 2½ cm (1 in) border.

3 Sprinkle the cheese over the top.
Lay a second tortilla on top of the
filling and press all the way round.

4 Brush a large frying pan with half the
oil. Lay the quesadillas in the pan
one at a time. Cook for 1 minute.
Turn and cook the other side until
the cheese is melted, adding the
remaining oil if they begin to stick.

Per serving		% energy
Energy	532 kcal	
Protein	22 g	17%
Fat	15 g	26%
Carbohydrate	82 g	57%
Fibre	8.2 g	

HEALTHY FAST FOOD

In this chapter, popular fast foods such as burgers and pizzas have been given a subtle makeover to substantially reduce their fat content and boost their nutritional value. Not only do they taste good but they really are fun to make!

SPICY CHICKEN FILLET BURGERS

10 minutes to prepare!

Makes 4 burgers

4 boneless chicken breast fillets
2 tsp oil
I tsp each of cumin, coriander and paprika
Pinch of chilli powder
4 wholemeal baps
Lettuce, tomato and low calorie salad dressing

1 Lightly rub the chicken fillets in the oil.
2 Mix together the spices in a shallow dish. Add the chicken to the spice mixture and toss to coat.

3 Cook the chicken in a non-stick pan over a high heat for about 3–4 minutes each side until tender and cooked through.
4 Toast the cut side of the baps. Place a chicken fillet, lettuce, tomatoes and dressing in each bap.

Per serving (excluding salad garnish)		% energy
Energy	285 kcal	
Protein	25 g	35%
Fat	6.8 g	21%
Carbohydrate	34 g	44%
Fibre	4.1 g	

GRILLED CHICKEN BURGERS

Low in fat and high in protein

Makes 4 servings

350 g (12 oz) lean minced chicken
50 g (2 oz) fresh breadcrumbs
½ small onion, finely chopped
2 tbsp fresh (or 1 tbsp dried)
herbs, e.g. parsley, thyme
Salt and freshly ground pepper to
taste
4 tbsp low fat salad dressing
1 tsp mustard
4 baps
Tomato slices

1 In a bowl, combine the chicken,
breadcrumbs, onion, fresh herbs and
seasoning. Mix until well blended.
Shape into 4 equal patties
approximately 1½ cm (½ in) thick.

2 Heat a non-stick pan over a
medium-high heat. Dry fry the
burgers 5–6 minutes on each side
until browned on the outside and
no longer pink in the centre.

3 Mix together the salad dressing and
mustard.

4 Place the burgers in baps with the
tomato slices and sauce.

Per serving (excluding salad garnish)		% energy
Energy	347 kcal	
Protein	27 g	31%
Fat	6.9 g	18%
Carbohydrate	47 g	51%
Fibre	4.7 g	

FISH BURGERS

These burgers are good made with plaice, cod or coley.

Makes 4 burgers

4 white fish fillets (approx. 75 g/
3 oz each)
2 tsp oil
4 wholemeal baps
Lettuce leaves, cucumber slices
1 tbsp reduced fat mayonnaise
2 tbsp plain yoghurt
1 tbsp chopped chives
Freshly ground black pepper

1 Cook the fish fillets in the oil over a
high heat for about 2–3 minutes
each side, or until the fish flakes
easily when tested with a fork.

2 Toast the baps.

3 Combine the mayonnaise, yoghurt
and chives.

4 Place a fish fillet, lettuce and
cucumber on the bottom half of
each bap. Place a spoonful of
mayonnaise dressing on top of the
fish, season to taste with pepper
and replace the top of the bap.

Per serving (excluding salad garnish)		% energy
Energy	297 kcal	
Protein	25 g	33%
Fat	7.2 g	22%
Carbohydrate	36 g	45%
Fibre	4.1 g	

LEAN HAMBURGERS

Homemade burgers contain none of the processed fat, flavour enhancers and salt found in most ready made versions.

Makes 4 burgers

350 g (12 oz) extra-lean minced
meat
3 tbsp water
½ small onion, chopped
2 tbsp parsley
Freshly ground black pepper
4 wholemeal baps
Shredded lettuce, sliced tomato,
grated carrot

1 Place the minced meat, water,
   onion, parsley and pepper in a bowl.
   Mix well to combine.

2 Divide the mixture into 4 patties.
   Dry fry in a hot non-stick pan or
   over a barbecue for 3–4 minutes
   each side.

3 Place lettuce, tomato and carrots on
   the bottom half of each bap, top
   with a burger and replace the top of
   the bap.

Per serving (excluding salad garnish)		% energy
Energy	281 kcal	
Protein	24 g	35%
Fat	6.1 g	19%
Carbohydrate	35 g	46%
Fibre	4.4 g	

SPICY LENTIL BURGERS

Makes 4 burgers

1 tbsp oil
1 onion, finely chopped
1 tbsp curry powder
175 g (6 oz) red lentils
600 ml (1 pint)
vegetable stock
100 g (4 oz) fresh
wholemeal breadcrumbs
Salt and freshly ground black
pepper to taste
A little oil for brushing
4 wholemeal baps
Salad leaves
4 tbsp Greek yoghurt mixed with
a pinch of curry powder

High in fibre, protein and iron

1 Heat the oil in a large pan and cook
   the onion until softened. Stir in the
   curry powder and cook for a
   further 3 minutes.

2 Add the lentils and stock. Bring to
   the boil and simmer for 20–25
   minutes. Alternatively, cook in a
   pressure cooker for 3 minutes and
   turn off the heat.

3 Allow to cool slightly and mix in the
   breadcrumbs. Shape into 4 burgers.

4 Place on a lightly-oiled baking tray
   and brush with a little oil.

5 Bake for 7–10 minutes at
   200°C/400°F/gas mark 6 until golden
   and firm.

6 Split the baps and place one burger
   inside each, together with salad
   leaves and a tablespoon of yoghurt
   sauce.

Per serving (excluding salad garnish)		% energy
Energy	449 kcal	
Protein	21 g	18%
Fat	6 g	12%
Carbohydrate	84 g	70%
Fibre	7.2 g	

HEALTHY FAST FOOD

203

BEAN BURGERS

You can use any type of beans for this recipe, as all are high in protein, fibre, iron and B vitamins.

Makes 4 burgers

1 tin (420 g) beans, drained, e.g. black eye beans, red kidney beans, butter beans, cannelini beans
1 tbsp oil
1 onion, chopped
1 celery stick
2 garlic cloves, crushed
1 tbsp curry powder
2 tbsp tomato purée
25 g (1 oz) fresh breadcrumbs
Salt and freshly ground black pepper
4 wholemeal baps
Salad leaves, sliced tomato
4 tbsp plain yoghurt

1 Purée the beans in a food processor.
2 Heat the oil in a pan and fry the onion and celery until softened. Add the garlic and curry powder and cook for 1 minute.
3 Mix together the beans with the fried vegetables and tomato purée, mash them well then season with salt and pepper.
4 Shape into 4 burgers and coat with breadcrumbs.
5 Brush a non-stick pan with a little oil and cook the burgers for approximately 3 minutes each side until golden.
6 Split and toast the baps and sandwich around the bean burgers, salad leaves, tomato and a spoonful of yoghurt.

Per serving (excluding salad garnish)		% energy
Energy	331 kcal	
Protein	15 g	19%
Fat	5.6 g	15%
Carbohydrate	59 g	66%
Fibre	7.9 g	

BASIC PIZZA

This can be made in a bread maker using the 'pizza' or 'dough' mode, follow the instructions in the manufacturer's booklet.

Makes 1 large pizza

Base:
225 g (8 oz) strong white flour
½ sachet easy-blend yeast
½ tsp salt
175 ml (6 fl oz) warm water
1 tbsp olive oil
Topping:
See page 206

1 Mix the flour, yeast and salt in a large bowl.
2 Make a well in the centre and add the oil and half the water. Stir with a wooden spoon, gradually adding more liquid until you have a pliable dough.
3 Turn the dough out onto a floured surface and knead for about 5 minutes until you have a smooth and elastic dough.
4 Place the dough in a clean, lightly-oiled bowl, cover with a tea towel and leave in a warm place for about 1 hour or until doubled in size (go and have a workout!).
5 Knock down the dough and knead briefly before rolling out on a surface to the desired shape.
6 Transfer to an oiled pizza dish or baking tray and finish shaping by hand. The dough should be approximately 5 mm (¼ in) thick. For a thicker crust, let the dough rise for another 30 minutes. The pizza is now ready for topping (see page 206) and baking.
7 Bake on the top shelf of the oven at 220°C/425°F/gas mark 7 for 15–20 minutes or until the topping is bubbling and the crust golden brown.

Per serving (¼ pizza)		% energy
Energy	297 kcal	
Protein	13 g	17%
Fat	8.1 g	25%
Carbohydrate	46 g	58%
Fibre	2.6 g	

QUICK PIZZA

This scone base has a wonderfully light and crumbly texture.

Makes I large pizza

Base:
  225 g (8 oz) self raising white flour
  1 tsp baking powder
  ½ tsp salt
  40 g (1½ oz) butter or margarine
  150 ml (5 fl oz) skimmed milk
Topping:
  See page 206

1 Mix the flour, baking powder and salt in a bowl.

2 Rub in the butter or margarine until the mixture resembles breadcrumbs.

3 Add the milk, quickly mixing with a fork until the mixture comes together.

4 Roll or press the dough into a circle approx. 25 cm (10 in) in diameter and transfer onto a baking tray or pizza pan.

5 The base is now ready for topping. Bake at 220°C/425°F/gas mark 7 for 15 minutes.

Variations

If you don't have time to make your own pizza base, use any of the following:

• ready-made chilled or frozen pizza base

• foccacia bread, halved horizontally

• ciabatta loaf, halved horizontally

• wholemeal or white pitta bread

• English muffins, toasted and split horizontally

• French bread, halved horizontally

Per serving (¼ pizza)		% energy
Energy	352 kcal	
Protein	13 g	15%
Fat	13 g	34%
Carbohydrate	48 g	51%
Fibre	2.6 g	

205

CHEESE AND TOMATO PIZZA

Tomato sauce:
300 ml (½ pint) passata (smooth
sieved tomatoes) or chopped
tinned tomatoes or ready-made
pasta sauce
1 tbsp tomato purée
2 tbsp fresh chopped herbs or 1
tbsp dried basil
Half an onion, very thinly sliced
100 g (4 oz) mozzarella

1 Mix together the passata, chopped
tomatoes or sauce, tomato purée
and herbs.
2 Spread on top of the pizza base.
Scatter over the onions, the grated
cheese and any additional toppings
from the list below.
3 Bake at 220°C/425°F/gas mark 7 for
15–20 minutes until the cheese is
bubbling and golden brown.

Pizza Toppings

Add any combination of the following:

• sliced raw vegetables, e.g. tomatoes,
mushrooms, peppers, courgettes,
asparagus, leeks
• well-drained, cooked spinach
• broccoli florets, cooked
• sweetcorn
• olives and sun dried tomatoes
• toasted sunflower seeds or pine
nuts
• thinly sliced tinned artichoke hearts
• flaked tinned tuna
• colourful cheeses, e.g. Red Leicester
or Double Gloucester
• strong flavoured cheeses, e.g.
parmesan, blue-veined cheese, extra
mature Cheddar cheese or feta
cheese
• pesto sauce

CALZONE

*This is really a folded pizza pie and is
great for wrapping and eating on the
run as there are no messy toppings to
worry about.*

Makes 1 calzone

Dough:
225 g (8 oz) strong white flour
½ sachet easy blend yeast
½ tsp salt
175 ml (6 fl oz) warm water
1 tbsp oil
Filling:
200 ml (7 fl oz) passata (smooth
sieved tomatoes) or tinned
chopped tomatoes
1 tbsp tomato purée
1 tbsp fresh or 1½ tsp dried mixed
herbs
Your choice of vegetables, e.g.
chopped onion, mushrooms,
peppers, broccoli florets
75 g (3 oz) grated cheese of your
choice

1 Mix the flours, yeast and salt in a
large bowl.
2 Make a well in the centre and add the
oil and half the water. Stir with a
wooden spoon, gradually adding more
liquid until you have a pliable dough.
3 Turn the dough out onto a floured
surface. Knead, adding a little more
flour if necessary until you have a
smooth, elastic, not-too-sticky
dough. This should take 5–10
minutes.
4 Place the dough in a clean lightly-
oiled bowl, cover with a tea towel
and leave in a warm place for
approximately 1 hour, or until
doubled in size.
5 Punch down the dough and knead
briefly.
6 Roll out the dough into a large
circle. Dampen the outside rim with
a little water.

7 Mix together the passata or chopped tomatoes, tomato purée and herbs. Spread over the circle leaving a 2 cm gap around the outside.

8 Pile the vegetables and cheese on one half of the circle. Fold the circle in half and press the edges firmly together. Brush with milk.

9 Place on a baking sheet and bake at 220°C/425°F/gas mark 7 for 15–20 minutes.

Per serving (¼ calzone, excluding vegetables)		% energy
Energy	321 kcal	
Protein	13 g	16%
Fat	11 g	31%
Carbohydrate	46 g	53%
Fibre	2.3 g	

23

SNACK BARS AND COOKIES

Home-made snack bars and cookies are far cheaper than commercial varieties and, in most cases, lower in fat and higher in important nutrients. These recipes make use of highly nutritious ingredients such as oats and other cereals, dried fruit and nuts. They also make ideal snacks for eating on the run.

MUESLI BARS

Try to use the no-added sugar muesli for this recipe.

Makes 12 bars

175 g (6 oz) oats
75 g (3 oz) muesli
150 g (5 oz) dried fruit mixture,
e.g. raisins, dates, apricots, figs,
apple, pineapple
3 heaped tbsp honey
2 egg whites
175 ml (6 fl oz) apple juice

1 Combine the oats, muesli and dried fruit in a bowl.

2 Warm the honey in a small saucepan until it is runny. Add to the bowl.

3 Stir in the remaining ingredients.

4 Press the mixture into a lightly-oiled 18 × 28 cm (7 × 11 in) baking tin. Bake at 180°C/350°F/gas mark 4 for 20–25 minutes until golden. When cool, cut into bars.

Per serving (1 bar)		% energy
Energy	141 kcal	
Protein	3.4 g	10%
Fat	1.9 g	12%
Carbohydrate	30 g	78%
Fibre	1.9 g	

OATY FRUIT BARS

An ideal post-workout snack, these bars are practically fat-free and are a great source of iron, vitamin A (beta-carotene) and carbohydrates.

Makes 16 bars

175 g (6 oz) porridge oats
175 g (6 oz) plain white or wholemeal flour
175 g (6 oz) Demerara sugar
1 tsp mixed spice
225 g (8 oz) prunes puréed with 6 tbsp water
1 egg white
100 g (4 oz) dried apricots
100 g (4 oz) sultanas
225 ml (8 fl oz) orange juice

1 Place the oats, flour, sugar, spice, prune purée and egg white in a large bowl. Combine with a fork or with your hands until you have a rough crumbly mixture.

2 Cook the apricots, sultanas and orange juice in a saucepan for 5 minutes, or until the liquid has been absorbed.

3 Mix the fruit with the oat mixture.

4 Spoon into a 26 × 17 cm (10 × 7 in) baking tin. Bake at 180°C/350°F/gas mark 4 for 35–40 minutes, until firm and crisp on the surface. When cool, cut into bars.

Per serving (1 bar)		% energy
Energy	186 kcal	
Protein	3.6 g	8%
Fat	1.3 g	6%
Carbohydrate	43 g	86%
Fibre	2.7 g	

DATE AND WALNUT BARS

Walnuts are rich in essential fatty acids, necessary for good athletic performance.

Makes 12 bars

225 g (8 oz) wholemeal self raising flour
1 tsp cinnamon
2 tbsp oil
75 g (3 oz) brown sugar
1 large egg
200 ml (7 fl oz) skimmed milk
175 g (6 oz) chopped dates
50 g (2 oz) chopped walnuts

1 Place the first six ingredients in a bowl and mix together.

2 Stir in the dates and walnuts.

3 Spoon the mixture into a lightly-oiled shallow 18 × 28 cm (7 × 11 in) baking tin.

4 Bake at 180°C/350°F/gas mark 4 for 20–25 minutes, until golden brown. When cool, cut into bars.

Per serving (1 bar)		% energy
Energy	189 kcal	
Protein	4.8 g	10%
Fat	6.3 g	30%
Carbohydrate	30 g	60%
Fibre	2.5 g	

FRUIT AND NUT BARS

These bars are packed with vitamins and minerals, as well as essential fats from the nuts and seeds.

Makes 12 bars

50 g (2 oz) margarine or butter
3 heaped tbsp honey
2 x 125 g cartons plain yoghurt
225 g (8 oz) low fat soft cheese or
cottage cheese
4 egg whites
50 g (2 oz) chopped nuts, e.g.
almonds, walnuts, brazils
75 g (3 oz) sultanas
225 g (8 oz) wholemeal self raising
flour
50 ml (2 fl oz) skimmed milk
Optional:
25 g (1 oz) sunflower or pumpkin
seeds/40 g (1½ oz) desiccated
coconut/50 g (2 oz) dried
apricots/50 g (2 oz) chopped figs

1 Combine the margarine or butter,
honey, yoghurt and soft cheese.

2 Beat in the eggs.

3 Stir in the remaining ingredients.
Add extra milk if the mixture seems
dry.

4 Spoon the mixture into a lightly-oiled
18 × 28 cm (7 × 11 in) baking tin.

5 Bake at 160°C/325°F/gas mark 3 for
35–40 minutes, until firm and
golden brown. When cool, cut into
bars.

APRICOT BARS

Apricots are rich in beta-carotene, a powerful antioxidant

Makes 8 bars

100 g (4 oz) dried apricots
6 tbsp orange juice
100 g (4 oz) self raising white flour
50 g (2 oz) sugar
2 eggs
100 g (4 oz) sultanas

1 Blend the apricots and juice
together in a food processor until
smooth.

2 Mix together the flour and sugar in
a bowl.

3 Add the apricot purée, eggs and
sultanas. Mix together.

4 Spoon the mixture into a 7 in
square cake tin. Bake at
180°C/350°F/gas mark 4 for 30–35
minutes, until golden brown. When
cool, cut into bars.

Per serving (1 bar)		% energy
Energy	152 kcal	
Protein	6.3 g	17%
Fat	6.2 g	36%
Carbohydrate	19 g	47%
Fibre	1.7 g	

Per serving (1 bar)		% energy
Energy	155 kcal	
Protein	3.9 g	10%
Fat	1.9 g	11%
Carbohydrate	33 g	79%
Fibre	1.1 g	

SNACK BARS AND COOKIES

RAISIN SCONES

The secret to making light scones is to mix the dough very quickly and handle it as little as possible. These scones make a nutritious, low fat, sweet snack.

Makes 10 bars

100 g (4 oz) wholemeal self raising flour
100g (4 oz) self raising white flour
1 tsp baking powder
¼ tsp salt
½ tsp cinnamon
50 g (2 oz) butter
40 g (1½ oz) sugar
50 g (2 oz) raisins
175 ml (6 fl oz) skimmed milk

Great for refuelling after a workout

1 In a large bowl, mix together the flours, baking powder, salt and cinnamon.
2 Roughly chop the butter and rub into the flour mixture with your fingertips until it resembles breadcrumbs. Alternatively, mix in a food processor.
3 Stir in the sugar and raisins.
4 Add the milk gradually, mixing quickly with a fork until it forms a soft dough. Do not over mix.
5 Press the dough to a thickness of about 1½ cm (½ in) on a floured surface. Cut into approximately 10 rounds using a scone cutter.
6 Transfer onto a lightly-oiled baking tray, brush with milk, and bake at 200°C/400°F/gas mark 6 for 10 minutes, or until lightly browned on top.

Variations

- Apricot Scones: replace the raisins with 50 g (2 oz) chopped, dried, ready to eat apricots. Omit the cinnamon.
- Cheese Scones: replace the sugar, cinnamon and raisins with 50 g (2 oz) grated Cheddar cheese.

- Walnut Scones: replace the raisins with 50 g (2 oz) chopped walnuts.

Per serving (1 scone)		% energy
Energy	162 kcal	
Protein	3.4 g	9%
Fat	5.4 g	29%
Carbohydrate	27 g	62%
Fibre	1.6 g	

FRUIT COOKIES

Low in fat, packed with fibre, iron and protein

Makes 20 bars

225 g (8 oz) wholemeal self raising flour
40 g (1½ oz) brown sugar
75 g (3 oz) dried fruit
2 tbsp oil
3 egg whites
4–5 tbsp skimmed milk

1 Combine the flour, sugar and fruit in a bowl.
2 Stir in the oil, egg whites and milk and lightly mix into a stiff dough.
3 Place spoonfuls of the mixture onto a lightly-oiled baking tray.
4 Bake at 180°C/350°F/gas mark 4 for 12–15 minutes, until golden brown.

Variations

- Fruit & Nut Cookies: add 50 g (2 oz) chopped walnuts or almonds.
- Peanut Cookies: replace dried fruit with 2 tbsp peanut butter.
- Muesli Cookies: substitute 75 g (3 oz) of the flour with the same weight of muesli.
- Sunflower Cookies: replace fruit with 50 g (2 oz) sunflower seeds.

Per serving (1 cookie)		% energy
Energy	67 kcal	
Protein	2 g	12%
Fat	1.4 g	18%
Carbohydrate	12 g	70%
Fibre	1.1 g	

OATMEAL COOKIES

Makes 20 bars

4 tbsp margarine or butter
75 g (3 oz) brown sugar
2 eggs
1 tsp vanilla essence
150 g (5 oz) porridge oats
75 g (3 oz) white flour
¼ tsp baking powder
¼ tsp cinnamon
50 g (2 oz) raisins

Perfect for refuelling after working out

1 Mix together the margarine or butter and sugar until light and fluffy.

2 Beat in the eggs and vanilla.

3 Add the remaining ingredients and mix until just combined. You should have a fairly stiff mixture.

4 Place spoonfuls onto a lightly-oiled baking sheet.

5 Bake at 180°C/350°F/gas mark 4 for 10 minutes, or until golden brown.

Variations

• Coconut Oatmeal Cookies: replace raisins with the same weight of desiccated coconut.

• Pecan Oatmeal Cookies: replace raisins with the same weight of chopped pecan nuts.

Per serving (1 cookie)		% energy
Energy	91 kcal	
Protein	2.1 g	9%
Fat	3 g	30%
Carbohydrate	15 g	61%
Fibre	0.7 g	

APPLE SAUCE COOKIES

A good way of getting extra fruit in your diet

Makes 20 bars

50 g (2 oz) butter or margarine
100 g (4 oz) brown sugar
1 large egg
250 ml (8 fl oz) apple sauce
175 g (6 oz) self raising white flour
½ tsp cinnamon
¼ tsp nutmeg
Optional:
50 g (2 oz) currants
40 g (1½ oz) chopped walnuts

1 Mix together the butter or margarine and brown sugar in a large bowl.

2 Add the egg and apple sauce and mix together until smooth.

3 Add flour, cinnamon and nutmeg and mix well.

4 Stir in the currants and walnuts.

5 Place heaped teaspoons of the mixture onto a lightly-oiled baking tray.

6 Bake at 190°C/375°F/gas mark 5 for 8–10 minutes, until firm to the touch.

Per serving (1 cookie)		% energy
Energy	92 kcal	
Protein	1.3 g	6%
Fat	2.9 g	28%
Carbohydrate	16 g	66%
Fibre	0.5 g	

24 PUDDINGS AND DESSERTS

Puddings and desserts can make a substantial contribution to the nutritional value of your meal. They are a superb way of getting extra fruit, extra milk or extra yoghurt into your daily diet. The following recipes contain significantly less fat than traditional puddings so you can confidently include them in your eating plans.

RAISIN CHEESECAKE

Makes 8 large slices

Base:
  25 g (1 oz) butter
  1 tbsp golden syrup (or honey)
  100 g (4 oz) ginger biscuits, crushed
Filling:
  75 g (3 oz) raisins
  3 tbsp dark rum
  450 g (1 lb) cottage cheese or quark
  75 g (3 oz) soft light brown sugar
  2 eggs
  1½ tbsp cornflour

1 To make the base, melt together the butter and syrup. Stir in the biscuit crumbs then press into the base of a 20 cm (8 in) springform or cheesecake tin.

2 Soak the raisins in the rum, ideally for half an hour (or as long as you can).

3 Blend the remaining ingredients in a liquidiser or food processor until smooth. Alternatively, sieve the cottage cheese and beat the ingredients together in a bowl.

4 Stir in the raisins and rum.

5 Pour the filling into the tin.

6 Bake at 180°C/350°F/gas mark 4 for 45 minutes. Turn off the oven and slightly open the door. Leave the cheesecake to cool in the oven until it reaches room temperature. Place the cheesecake in the fridge.

Per serving (1 slice)		% energy
Energy	272 kcal	
Protein	11 g	16%
Fat	8.8 g	29%
Carbohydrate	37 g	55%
Fibre	0.4 g	

BAKED LEMON CHEESECAKE (BASIC RECIPE)

This is my favourite dessert and one I shall never tire of making or eating. This low fat version of the baked cheesecake takes only minutes to prepare and can be infinitely varied according to the fresh or tinned fruit you have available. It is low in fat and a good source of protein, calcium and vitamins. (It is well worth investing in a cheesecake tin if you don't already have one.)

Makes 8 large slices

Base:
100 g (4 oz) digestive biscuits, crushed into crumbs
25 g (1 oz) butter
1 heaped tbsp honey

Filling:
450 g (1 lb) cottage cheese (or quark)
75 g (3 oz) sugar
2 eggs
Grated rind and juice of 1 lemon
150 ml (¼ pint) low fat plain yoghurt
1 tbsp cornflour
100 g (4 oz) sultanas

1 To make the base, melt the butter and honey together then stir in the biscuit crumbs. Press into the base of a 20 cm (8 in) springform or cheesecake tin.

2 To make the filling, blend all the ingredients except the sultanas in a liquidiser or food processor until smooth. Alternatively, sieve the cottage cheese then beat the ingredients together in a mixing bowl.

3 Stir in the sultanas and pour into the tin.

4 Bake at 180°C/350°F/gas mark 4 for 45 minutes. Turn off the oven and slightly open the door. Leave the cheesecake to cool in the oven until it reaches room temperature. Place the cheesecake in the fridge; the flavour actually improves if it has been refrigerated overnight.

Variations

• Apricot: add 100 g (4 oz) puréed cooked dried apricots to the mixture. Omit the lemon and sultanas.

• Apple Spice: add 1 large grated cooking apple and 1 tsp cinnamon to the mixture.

• Vanilla: substitute 1 tsp vanilla extract for the lemon.

• Banana: add 2 mashed ripe bananas to the mixture. Omit the sultanas.

• Pineapple: add 1 tin (200 g) of pineapple (finely chopped) to the mixture. Omit the lemon and sultanas.

• Mango: add 1 tin (400 g) mango (well drained and mashed) to the mixture. Omit the lemon and sultanas.

• Raspberry: add 225 g (8 oz) fresh or frozen raspberries and omit lemon and sultanas.

• Blackcurrant: add 4 tbsp blackcurrant conserve or jam.

• Date and Walnut: stir in 75 g (3 oz) chopped dates and 50 g (2 oz) chopped walnuts. Omit lemon and sultanas.

• Spicy Apple: add 2 grated apples and 1 tsp cinnamon. Omit the sultanas.

• Peanut and Raisin: add 2 heaped tbsp crunchy peanut butter and 50 g (2 oz) raisins.

• Strawberry: add 4 tbsp strawberry pure fruit spread to the filling and top with 100 g (4 oz) fresh sliced strawberries.

• Chocolate: add 100 g (4 oz) melted milk or plain chocolate.

PUDDINGS AND DESSERTS

Per serving (1 slice)		% energy
Energy	293 kcal	
Protein	12 g	16%
Fat	9.9 g	30%
Carbohydrate	42 g	54%
Fibre	0.7 g	

CHOCOLATE COOKIE CHEESECAKE

Heavenly and indulgent, but surprisingly much healthier than it sounds!

Makes 8 slices

Base:
25 g (1 oz) butter
1 tbsp golden syrup or honey
100 g (4 oz) chocolate bourbon biscuits, crushed

Filling:
450 g (1 lb) cottage cheese
75 g (3 oz) sugar
2 eggs
150 ml (¼ pint) thick plain yoghurt
100 g (4 oz) chocolate bourbon biscuits, coarsely broken into small pieces
3 tbsp half fat crème fraîche
Chocolate curls or flakes

1 To make the base, melt the butter and syrup or honey. Stir in the biscuits and press into the base of a 20 cm (8 in) springform or cheesecake tin.

2 To make the filling, place the cottage cheese, sugar, eggs and yoghurt in a food processor or liquidiser and blend until smooth.

3 Pour half of this filling into the tin.

4 Top with the broken biscuits.

5 Cover with the remaining filling mixture.

6 Bake at 180°C/350°F/gas mark 4 for 45 minutes. Turn off the oven and slightly open the door. Leave the cheesecake to cool in the oven until it reaches room temperature. Spread the half fat crème fraîche over the cheesecake and sprinkle with the chocolate curls or flake. Place the cheesecake in the fridge.

Per serving (1 slice)		% energy
Energy	313 kcal	
Protein	13 g	17%
Fat	13 g	37%
Carbohydrate	39 g	46%
Fibre	0 g	

CRUNCHY APPLE CRUMBLE

This dessert will help restock your glycogen stores. The oats and apples both have a low glycaemic index so you'll get a sustained energy release. It is also a delicious way of adding lots of fruit to your diet.

Makes 4 servings

700 g (1½ lb) eating apples, sliced
50 g (2 oz) raisins
½ tsp cinnamon
50 g (2 oz) plain flour
50 g (2 oz) low fat spread
50 g (2 oz) porridge oats
40 g (1½ oz) brown sugar
25 g (1 oz) toasted almonds, chopped (alternatively use walnuts/pecans/hazelnuts)

1 Place the apples, raisins and cinnamon in a deep baking dish. Combine well and add 3–4 tbsp water.
2 For the topping, combine the flour and low fat spread in a food processor (or rub in by hand).
3 Stir in the remaining ingredients. Sprinkle over the apples.
4 Bake at 190°C/375°C/gas mark 5 for 20–25 minutes.

Variations

Substitute 700 g (1½ lb) of prepared fruit for the apples. Try the following:

- chopped rhubarb and 40 g (1½ oz) sugar
- fresh or tinned apricots
- pears and raspberries
- fresh or frozen summer fruits, e.g. blackcurrants, raspberries, strawberries
- pears and bananas
- blackberries and apples

Per serving		% energy
Energy	312 kcal	
Protein	5.6 g	7%
Fat	5.2 g	15%
Carbohydrate	65 g	78%
Fibre	5.4 g	

FRUIT RICE PUDDING

This super quick, high carbohydrate pudding is an excellent way of refuelling after exercise, and of sneaking extra fresh fruit into your diet.

Makes 2 servings

1 tin (400 g) low fat rice pudding
225 g (8 oz) colourful fruit, e.g. raspberries, blackberries, blueberries
150 ml (5 fl oz) low fat fruit yoghurt, e.g. raspberry

1 Combine the rice pudding, fruit and yoghurt in a dish.
2 Spoon into individual bowls.

Variations

- You could use any of the following fresh or tinned fruits in place of the berries: peach, apricot, pineapple, mango and a complementary flavoured yoghurt.

Per serving		% energy
Energy	282 kcal	
Protein	13 g	18%
Fat	1.3 g	4%
Carbohydrate	59 g	78%
Fibre	3 g	

HOT WINTER FRUIT SALAD

Experiment with dried apples, pears or peaches – all rich in fibre and iron.

Makes 4 servings

100 g (4 oz) dried fruit mixture
250 ml (8 fl oz) orange juice
1 ruby grapefruit, segmented
1 orange, segmented
1 pear, chopped

1 Place the dried fruit and orange juice into a pan and bring to the boil. Simmer for 5 minutes.
2 Add the remaining fruit.
3 Serve with low fat yoghurt.

Per serving		% energy
Energy	121 kcal	
Protein	2.2 g	7%
Fat	0.3 g	2%
Carbohydrate	29 g	91%
Fibre	3.6 g	

COOL SUMMER FRUIT SALAD

Make a larger quantity – it will keep in the fridge for up to two days.

Makes 4 servings

100 g (4 oz) strawberries
100 g (4 oz) grapes
4 kiwi fruit, sliced
4 apricots, chopped
150 ml (5 fl oz) tropical fruit juice

1 Combine the prepared fruit and fruit juice in a bowl.
2 Spoon into individual bowls and serve with very low fat fromage frais.

Per serving		% energy
Energy	167 kcal	
Protein	3.1 g	8%
Fat	0.6 g	3%
Carbohydrate	40 g	89%
Fibre	5.4 g	

BANANA BREAD PUDDING

This healthy version of bread pudding is low in fat and high in potassium and fibre.

10 slices wholemeal bread
2 bananas, sliced
50 g (2 oz) sugar
3 eggs
900 ml (1½ pints) skimmed milk
Cinnamon

1 Trim the crusts from the bread and cut into quarters diagonally.
2 Arrange one third of the bread triangles in a lightly greased baking dish.
3 Arrange one sliced banana on top and then repeat the layers with the remaining bread and banana, finishing with the bread.
4 Combine the sugar, eggs, and milk. Pour over the bread then sprinkle with cinnamon.
5 If you have time, allow to stand for 30 minutes.
6 Bake at 180°C/350°F/gas mark 4 for 40 minutes, or until the pudding is set and golden brown on top.

Per serving		% energy
Energy	437 kcal	
Protein	22 g	20%
Fat	7.5 g	16%
Carbohydrate	75 g	64%
Fibre	5.6 g	

PUDDINGS AND DESSERTS

LOW FAT ICE CREAM

This is really a cheat's ice cream as it is simplicity itself to make. The whisking incorporates a lot of air so all you need to do is put it in the freezer and wait – there is no stirring and refreezing. It is considerably lower in fat than standard ice cream, and is rich in protein, calcium and vitamin A. Adding extra fruit boosts the vitamin and fibre content.

Makes 4 large servings

250 ml (8 fl oz) evaporated milk, chilled in the fridge
50 g (2 oz) caster sugar
2 tsp vanilla essence

1 Pour the chilled milk into a bowl and whisk with an electric mixer for approximately 4 minutes, until thick and foamy and roughly tripled in volume.
2 Whisk in the sugar and vanilla until incorporated.
3 Pour the mixture into a shallow container and place in the freezer until frozen.

Variations

- Mango: purée the flesh of one large ripe mango and stir into the whisked milk. Omit the vanilla.
- Apricot: stir in 175 g (6 oz) puréed, soaked dried apricots and omit the vanilla.
- Raspberry: stir in 175 g (6 oz) mashed fresh or frozen raspberries and omit the vanilla.
- Blackcurrant or Blueberry: stir in 3 heaped tbsp blackcurrant or blueberry pure fruit spread. You may reduce the sugar by half.
- Hazelnut: stir in 50 g (2 oz) chopped toasted hazelnuts.
- Amaretto: stir in 1–2 tbsp amaretto (almond liqueur) and 50 g (2 oz) flaked toasted almonds. Omit the vanilla.

Per serving		% energy
Energy	153 kcal	
Protein	5.2 g	14%
Fat	5.9 g	34%
Carbohydrate	21 g	52%
Fibre	0 g	

APRICOT AND DATE BREAD PUDDING

This low fat adaptation of the classic pudding has a higher content of fibre, vitamin A and potassium.

Makes 4 servings

8 slices wholemeal bread, crusts trimmed
50 g (2 oz) dates, chopped
50 g (2 oz) dried apricots
2 eggs
2 tbsp honey
750 ml (1½ pints) skimmed/semi-skimmed milk
Pinch of cinnamon

1 Cut each slice of bread into diagonal quarters. Arrange one third of the triangles in a lightly-oiled 20 cm (8 in) square baking dish.
2 Sprinkle with half of the dates and apricots.
3 Place another layer of bread triangles on top. Sprinkle with the remaining dates and apricots and finish with a layer of the remaining bread.
4 Beat together the eggs, honey and milk. Pour over the pudding and sprinkle with the cinnamon.
5 Place the dish in a larger baking pan containing enough hot water to reach halfway up the sides of the dish. Bake at 180°C/350°F/gas mark 4 for 40 minutes, or until the pudding is just set and golden brown on top.

Per serving		% energy
Energy	354 kcal	
Protein	17 g	20%
Fat	5.4 g	14%
Carbohydrate	63 g	66%
Fibre	5.8 g	

FRUIT PANCAKES

Low in fat and high in fibre

Makes 4 servings

Batter:
50 g (2 oz) plain white flour
50 g (2 oz) plain wholemeal flour
2 eggs
300 ml (½ pint) skimmed milk
A little vegetable oil or oil spray
for frying
Filling:
225 g (8 oz) sliced fruit (see below)
200 g (7 oz) low fat vanilla fromage
frais

I Place all of the batter ingredients in
a liquidiser and blend until smooth.

2 Alternatively mix the flours in a
bowl. Make a well in the centre.
Beat the egg and milk and gradually
add to the flour, beating to make a
smooth batter.

3 Place a non-stick frying pan over a
high heat. Spray with oil spray or
add a few drops of oil.

4 Pour in enough batter to coat the
pan thinly and cook for 1–2 minutes
until golden brown on the underside.

5 Turn the pancake and cook the
other side for 30–60 seconds until
golden brown.

6 Turn out onto a plate, cover and
keep warm while you make the
other pancakes.

7 To make the filling, combine the
sliced fruit with the fromage frais.

8 Place spoonfuls of the fruit mixture
over one half of each pancake then
fold the pancakes into triangles.

Fruit suggestions: fresh strawberries,
sliced mango, tinned pineapple, fresh
or tinned apricots, sliced banana,
mixed berry fruits, tinned cherries,
sliced nectarines.

Per serving		% energy
Energy	209 kcal	
Protein	14 g	26%
Fat	4 g	17%
Carbohydrate	32 g	57%
Fibre	2.4 g	

PUDDINGS
AND DESSERTS

LOW FAT TIRAMISU

Both the fat and calorie content of this healthy pudding are a fraction of the classic Italian version. You can substitute fruit juice for the alcohol if you prefer.

Makes 4 servings

12 sponge fingers
100 ml (3½ fl oz) strong black coffee
1 tsp vanilla essence
1 tbsp Amaretto
1 tbsp brandy
450 g (1 lb) soft fruit, e.g. raspberries, blackberries, strawberries, tinned black cherries
225 g (8 oz) plain low fat fromage frais
225 g (8 oz) quark or ricotta cheese
2½ tbsp icing sugar, sifted
1 tbsp cocoa or chocolate powder

1 Line the bottom of a shallow baking dish with the sponge fingers.

2 Mix together the coffee, vanilla, Amaretto and brandy. Slowly sprinkle this mixture over the sponge fingers so that they evenly soak up all the liquid.

3 Place the fruit over the sponge fingers.

4 Combine the fromage frais, quark, and 2 tbsp of the icing sugar. Spread over the sponge fingers.

5 Combine the cocoa and the remaining icing sugar. Sift evenly over the surface of the pudding. Chill.

Per serving		% energy
Energy	244 kcal	
Protein	18 g	29%
Fat	3.1 g	11%
Carbohydrate	34 g	60%
Fibre	3.5 g	

BAKED BANANAS

One of the easiest desserts to make. It is high in carbohydrates, low in fat, and rich in potassium and magnesium. Topped with a little Greek yoghurt it is good enough to serve at dinner parties as well as for the family.

Makes 4 servings

4 large bananas
4 tbsp water
2 tbsp honey or maple syrup
½ tsp mixed spice
2 tbsp dark rum/50 g (2 oz) raisins/50 g (2 oz) chocolate buttons/1 tbsp lemon juice (all optional)

1 Chop the bananas into 2½ cm (1 in) chunks.

2 Place in a baking dish and combine with the remaining ingredients.

3 Bake at 200°C/400°F/gas mark 6 for 15 minutes, or microwave for 3 minutes.

Per serving		% energy
Energy	124 kcal	
Protein	1.2 g	4%
Fat	0.3 g	2%
Carbohydrate	31 g	94%
Fibre	1.1 g	

FRUIT CLAFOUTI

This French fruit custard is equally good eaten hot or cold. It is low in fat and is a good source of protein, vitamins and calcium.

Makes 4 servings

50 g (2 oz) plain white flour
50 g (2 oz) sugar
2 eggs
350 ml (12 fl oz) skimmed milk
450 g (1 lb) fruit, e.g. plums, tinned black cherries, raspberries, apples, tinned peaches
Pinch of nutmeg

1 Blend the flour, sugar, eggs and milk in a liquidiser. Alternatively, beat together by hand until smooth.
2 Place the fruit in the bottom of a shallow baking dish.
3 Pour in the batter and sprinkle the top with nutmeg.
4 Bake at 200°C/400°F/gas mark 6 for 40–45 minutes, until the custard is firm.

Per serving		% energy
Energy	221 kcal	
Protein	8.6 g	16%
Fat	3.6 g	15%
Carbohydrate	41 g	69%
Fibre	2.1 g	

YOGHURT AND FRUIT PUDDING

You can use frozen summer fruit or forest fruits if you prefer.

Makes 1 serving

1 carton (125 g or 150 g) low fat or virtually fat free fruit yoghurt
100 g (4 oz) fruit mixture, e.g. strawberries, blueberries, raspberries, peaches, bananas
Optional:
1 tbsp toasted flaked almonds/chopped hazelnuts

1 Spoon half of the yoghurt into a sundae glass (or small dish).
2 Top with half of the fruit followed by another layer of yoghurt.
3 Top with the remaining fruit and nuts (optional).

Per serving		% energy
Energy	169 kcal	
Protein	7.1 g	17%
Fat	1.1 g	6%
Carbohydrate	34 g	77%
Fibre	1.4 g	

OATMEAL AND RAISIN SCOTCH PANCAKES

A fantastic pudding which aids refuelling through slow release complex carbohydrates, protein and soluble fibre. These pancakes also double up as a nutritious snack that you can pop into your kit bag.

Makes 8 pancakes

2 large eggs
225 g (8 oz) cottage cheese
1 tbsp margarine or low fat spread
100 g (4 oz) oatmeal or porridge oats
75 g (3 oz) raisins or currants

1 Place the eggs, cottage cheese, margarine and oatmeal in a liquidiser and blend until smooth. Alternatively, beat together by hand in a bowl.

2 Add the raisins or currants and stir in carefully.

3 Lightly brush a non-stick frying pan with oil. Drop tablespoons of the batter onto the hot pan. When bubbles appear on the surface, flip over and cook for one more minute.

4 Serve with fresh fruit, puréed fruit or pure fruit spread.

Per serving (1 pancake)		% energy
Energy	146 kcal	
Protein	8 g	22%
Fat	4.6 g	28%
Carbohydrate	19 g	50%
Fibre	1.3 g	

COTTAGE CHEESE PANCAKES WITH BLUEBERRY SAUCE

Blueberries are rich in vitamin C and fibre. You could substitute them with other similar fruits, e.g. blackberries, blackcurrants or raspberries.

Makes 4 servings (8 pancakes)

Sauce:
225 g (8 oz) fresh or frozen blueberries
1 heaped tsp cornflour
2 tbsp honey
Pancakes:
225 g (8 oz) cottage cheese
175 g (6 oz) flour
3 eggs
175 ml (6 fl oz) semi-skimmed milk
1 tbsp sugar

1 Place the blueberries with 1 tbsp water in a saucepan and simmer for a few minutes until they burst.

2 Mix together the cornflour, honey and 3 tbsp water in a cup and add to the blueberries. Bring to the boil, stirring to thicken. Leave to cool.

3 In a bowl, combine the pancake ingredients.

4 Lightly brush or spray a thick-based frying pan with oil. Over a medium heat, drop spoonfuls of the pancake batter onto the hot pan. Cook for approximately 2 minutes, or until lightly browned on the underside. Flip and cook on the other side until lightly browned, about 1 minute.

5 Pile the pancakes onto a plate and spoon the blueberry sauce over the top.

Per serving		% energy
Energy	357 kcal	
Protein	20 g	22%
Fat	8.4 g	21%
Carbohydrate	54 g	57%
Fibre	3.1 g	

MUFFINS

Muffins are mini-cakes and these come with a lower fat content than the ordinary variety, which makes them ideal as portable healthy snacks. They are very easy to make, and the variations are almost infinite. If you plan to make them regularly, it's worth investing in a non-stick deep muffin (bun) tin. Muffins will keep for up to three days or, alternatively, freeze and defrost as you need them.

A word of warning: once you start making your own muffins you'll be hooked!

RAISIN MUFFINS

The perfect refuelling snack that no athlete should be without! You may use all wholemeal flour if you prefer but I find that a half and half mixture of white and wholemeal flour gives the lightest result.

Makes 12 muffins

100 g (4 oz) white self raising flour
100 g (4 oz) wholemeal self raising flour
Pinch of salt
40 g (1½ oz) soft brown sugar
1 tbsp oil
1 egg
200 ml (7 fl oz) skimmed milk
75 g (3 oz) raisins

1 Preheat the oven to 220°C/425°F/gas mark 7.
2 Mix the flours and salt together in a bowl.
3 Add the oil, sugar, egg and milk. Mix well.
4 Stir in the raisins.
5 Spoon into a non-stick muffin tray and bake for approximately 15 minutes until golden brown.

Variations

• Carrot and Nut: add 2 grated carrots and 50 g (2 oz) chopped walnuts or pecans. Omit the raisins.
• Blueberry: stir in 150 g (5 oz) fresh or 75 g (3 oz) dried blueberries instead of the raisins.
• Cherry: replace the raisins with 75 g (3 oz) halved glace cherries.

Per serving (1 muffin)		% energy
Energy	120 kcal	
Protein	3.6 g	12%
Fat	1.9 g	14%
Carbohydrate	24 g	74%
Fibre	1.4 g	

ORANGE MUFFINS

Good for breakfast on the run, they are high in carbohydrate and fibre, and low in fat.

Makes 16 muffins

2 eggs
75 g (3 oz) sugar
3 tbsp oil
200 ml (7 fl oz) skimmed milk
Grated rind and juice of 2 oranges
150 g (5 oz) self raising white flour
100 g (4 oz) wholemeal flour
½ tsp salt

1 Combine the eggs, sugar, oil, milk and rind and juice of the oranges in a bowl.
2 Combine the flours and salt in a bowl then fold into the wet mixture.
3 Spoon into lightly oiled muffin tins and bake at 200°C/400°F/gas mark 6 for 20 minutes.

Per serving (1 muffin)		% energy
Energy	112 kcal	
Protein	3.2 g	12%
Fat	3.2 g	25%
Carbohydrate	19 g	63%
Fibre	1.0 g	

CHOCOLATE CHIP MUFFINS

The perfect treat for chocoholics!

Makes 12 muffins

225 g (8 oz) self raising flour (half white/half wholemeal)
1 tsp baking powder
75 g (3 oz) sugar
40 g (1½ oz) cocoa, sieved
½ tsp salt
3 egg whites
3 tbsp oil
1 tsp vanilla essence
300 ml (½ pint) skimmed milk
50 g (2 oz) chocolate chips

1 Mix together the flour, baking powder, sugar, cocoa and salt in a large bowl.
2 Add the egg whites, oil, vanilla and milk and fold together. Add a little extra milk if necessary to produce a very soft mixture.
3 Fold the chocolate into the mixture.
4 Bake at 200°C/400°F/gas mark 6 for 20 minutes.

Per serving (1 muffin)		% energy
Energy	159 kcal	
Protein	4.4 g	11%
Fat	5.2 g	29%
Carbohydrate	25 g	60%
Fibre	1.7 g	

OATMEAL MUFFINS

Oats provide slow release complex carbohydrate thanks to their soluble fibre content.

Makes 12 muffins

175 g (6 oz) self raising flour (all white, or half wholemeal/half white)
100 g (4 oz) oats
100 g (4 oz) brown sugar
2 tsp baking powder
½ tsp salt
4 tbsp oil
1 tsp vanilla essence
1 large egg
225 ml (8 fl oz) skimmed milk or buttermilk
100 g (4 oz) fresh fruit or dried fruit (see variations)

1 In a large bowl, mix together the flour, oats, sugar, baking powder and salt.

2 Combine the oil, vanilla, egg and milk in a separate bowl then stir into the flour mixture.

3 Fold the fruit into the mixture.

4 Spoon the mixture into lightly oiled muffin tins, filling them two-thirds full.

5 Bake at 190°C/375°F/gas mark 5 for about 20 minutes until firm to the touch and light brown.

Variations

- Oatmeal Apple: add 100 g (4 oz) grated apples.
- Oatmeal Pineapple: add 100–175 g (4–6 oz) tinned chopped pineapple.
- Oatmeal Fig: add 75–100 g (3–4 oz) chopped dried figs.
- Oatmeal Blueberry: add 100 g (4 oz) fresh blueberries.
- Oatmeal Coconut: add 100 g (4 oz) shredded unsweetened coconut or desiccated coconut to the flour mixture.

Per serving (1 muffin)		% energy
Energy	188 kcal	
Protein	4.3 g	9%
Fat	5.5 g	26%
Carbohydrate	32 g	65%
Fibre	1.4 g	

BANANA MUFFINS

Take these in your kit bag for post workout refuelling.

Makes 12 muffins

2 large ripe bananas, mashed
75 g (3 oz) sugar
50 g (2 oz) butter
1 egg
100 ml (4 fl oz) skimmed milk
200 g (7 oz) self raising flour
Pinch of salt
½ tsp nutmeg
50 g (2 oz) chopped walnuts/50 g (2 oz) raisins (optional)

1 Mix together the bananas, sugar and butter.

2 Beat in the egg and milk.

3 Fold in the flour, salt, nutmeg and walnuts or raisins if applicable.

4 Spoon into a lightly oiled muffin tin and bake at 190°C/375°F/gas mark 5 for 20 minutes.

Per serving (1 muffin)		% energy
Energy	150 kcal	
Protein	2.7 g	7%
Fat	4.9 g	29%
Carbohydrate	25 g	64%
Fibre	0.7 g	

MUFFINS

CORN MUFFINS

Eat these savoury muffins for breakfast or for supper with a bowl of tomato soup. They are low in fat, and high in complex carbohydrate and fibre.

Makes 12 muffins

175 g (6 oz) cornmeal
1 tbsp baking powder
1 tsp salt
2 eggs
2 tbsp oil
250 g (9 oz) tin of creamed corn
250 ml (9 fl oz) plain yoghurt

1 Mix together the cornmeal, baking powder and salt in a large bowl.

2 In a separate bowl, combine the remaining ingredients.

3 Add the wet mixture to the cornmeal mixture and combine well.

4 Spoon into a lightly oiled muffin tin.

5 Bake at 200°C/400°F/gas mark 6 for 20 minutes until risen and golden.

See also breakfast muffins, page 191.

Per serving (1 muffin)		% energy
Energy	122 kcal	
Protein	4.3 g	14%
Fat	3.8 g	28%
Carbohydrate	18 g	58%
Fibre	0.6 g	

CAKES

This is a collection of my favourite low fat cake recipes, developed over several years and tested by many willing volunteers! Most make use of added fresh and dried fruit which boost the nutritional value as well as reducing the sugar and fat content. In fact, the following recipes are healthy enough to be regarded as everyday snacks instead of occasional treats.

BANANA CAKE

Bursting with vitamins, this high carbo-hydrate, fat-free snack should be a staple part of every athlete's diet.

Makes 12 slices

2 large ripe bananas
225 ml (8 fl oz) orange juice
300 g (10 oz) self raising flour (half wholemeal/half white)
100 g (4 oz) brown sugar
Pinch of salt
½ tsp each of mixed spice and cinnamon
2 egg whites
1 tbsp oil

1 Mash the bananas with the orange juice.

2 Mix together the flour, sugar, salt and spices in a bowl.

3 Add the banana juice mixture together with the egg whites and oil. Combine together.

4 Spoon into a lightly-oiled 2 lb loaf tin.

5 Bake at 160°C/325°F/gas mark 3 for about 1 hour. Check the cake is cooked by inserting a skewer or knife into the centre. It should come out clean.

Per serving (1 slice)		% energy
Energy	158 kcal	
Protein	3.5 g	9%
Fat	1.4 g	8%
Carbohydrate	35 g	83%
Fibre	1.8 g	

CAKES

APPLE CAKE

Less than
10 minutes
to prepare!

Makes 12 slices

3 eating apples, peeled
300 g (10 oz) self raising flour (half wholemeal/half white)
100 g (4 oz) brown sugar
1 tsp cinnamon
2 egg whites
100 ml (4 fl oz) apple juice

1 Grate the apples and place in a bowl with the remaining ingredients.

2 Mix together well.

3 Spoon into a lightly oiled loaf tin and bake at 160°C/325°F/gas mark 3 for about 1–1¼ hours. Check the cake is cooked by inserting a skewer or knife into the centre. It should come out clean.

CARROT CAKE

Traditional carrot cakes have a very high oil/fat and sugar content and are smothered in cream cheese. This low fat version is perfect for active people and tastes even better!

Makes 16 slices

225 g (8 oz) self raising flour (half wholemeal/half white)
Pinch of salt
2 tsp mixed spice
100 g (4 oz) brown sugar
3 carrots, grated
2 eating apples, grated
100 g (4 oz) sultanas or raisins
2 tbsp oil
175 ml (6 fl oz) orange or apple juice
2 egg whites

1 Mix together the flour, salt, spice and sugar in a bowl.

2 Stir in the carrots, apples and sultanas.

3 Add the oil, fruit juice and egg whites. Mix together well.

4 Spoon into a loaf tin or a 20 cm (8 in) round cake tin and bake at 160°C/325°F/gas mark 3 for about 1½ hours. Check the cake is cooked by inserting a skewer or knife into the centre. It should come out clean.

Per serving (1 slice)		% energy
Energy	98 kcal	
Protein	3.3 g	13%
Fat	0.5 g	4%
Carbohydrate	22 g	83%
Fibre	2 g	

Per serving (1 slice)		% energy
Energy	125 kcal	
Protein	2.2 g	7%
Fat	1.7 g	12%
Carbohydrate	27 g	81%
Fibre	1.5 g	

PUMPKIN CAKE

Make this cake in the autumn when pumpkins are plentiful and cheap. This low fat cake is surprisingly moist and moreish, and pumpkin is a terrific source of beta-carotene, potassium and fibre.

Makes 12 slices

225 g (8 oz) cooked mashed pumpkin
1 carton (125 g) low fat plain yoghurt
1 egg
100 g (4 oz) sugar
175 g (6 oz) self raising flour (or half wholemeal/half white)
1 tsp vanilla essence
75 g (3 oz) raisins

1 In a large bowl, mix together the pumpkin, yoghurt and egg.
2 Fold in the remaining ingredients.
3 Spoon the mixture into a lightly-oiled shallow 18 × 28 cm (7 × 11 in) baking tin.
4 Bake at 180°C/350°F/gas mark 4 for 35–40 minutes until firm and golden brown. Cut into slices.

Per serving (1 slice)		% energy
Energy	124 kcal	
Protein	2.7 g	9%
Fat	0.9 g	6%
Carbohydrate	28 g	85%
Fibre	0.8 g	

RAISIN CAKE

This cake is a staple food in my house!

Makes 8 squares

75 g (3 oz) raisins
100 ml (4 fl oz) orange juice
50 g (2 oz) sugar
50g (2 oz) low fat spread, melted
1 tsp vanilla essence
1 egg and 1 egg white
100 g (4 oz) self raising flour (wholemeal or white)
½ tsp cinnamon

1 Combine the raisins, orange juice, low fat spread, sugar and vanilla in a bowl.
2 Add the egg and egg white. Mix well.
3 Fold in the flour and cinnamon.
4 Spoon the mixture into a baking tin.
5 Bake at 180°C/350°F/gas mark 4 for about 15 minutes, until golden and firm to the touch. Cool and cut into squares.

Per serving (1 square)		% energy
Energy	154 kcal	
Protein	4 g	10%
Fat	4.2 g	25%
Carbohydrate	25 g	65%
Fibre	1.6 g	

CAKES

FRUIT CAKE

This cake is almost a complete meal – the dried fruit and nuts add valuable fibre, vitamins and minerals.

Makes 16 slices

225 g (8 oz) self raising flour (half wholemeal/half white)
75 g (3 oz) brown sugar
1 tsp cinnamon
2 eggs
4 tbsp oil
1 tsp vanilla
225 g (8 oz) dried fruit mixture (any combination of raisins, sultanas, currants, apricots, dates, pineapple, mango, apple, peaches, figs, papaya)
1 apple, grated
75 ml (3 fl oz) skimmed milk
Optional:
100 g (4 oz) chopped nuts of any variety/100 g (4 oz) grated courgettes/2 grated carrots/ 75 g (3 oz) glace cherries/grated lemon or orange rind

1 Mix together the flour, sugar, and cinnamon in a bowl.

2 Make a well in the centre and add the eggs, oil, vanilla, fruit and milk and any extra optional ingredients. Combine together well.

3 Spoon into a 23 cm (9 in) round or square baking tin and bake at 160°C/325°F/gas mark 3 for about 1¼–1½ hours. Check the cake is cooked by inserting a skewer or knife into the centre. It should come out clean.

Per serving (1 slice)		% energy
Energy	145 kcal	
Protein	2.9 g	8%
Fat	3.9 g	24%
Carbohydrate	26 g	68%
Fibre	1.2 g	

CHOCOLATE AND BANANA CAKE

Bananas and chocolate are a great combination and this recipe, thankfully, is low in fat too.

Makes 12 slices

2 ripe bananas, mashed
75 g (3 oz) brown sugar
3 tbsp oil
2 tsp vanilla essence
1 egg or 2 egg whites
1 carton (125 g) plain yoghurt
200 g (7 oz) self raising flour (half wholemeal/half white)
25 g (1 oz) cocoa powder, sieved
Pinch of salt
Optional:
50 g (2 oz) raisins/75 g (3 oz) chopped dates/50 g (2 oz) walnuts

1 Combine the bananas, sugar, oil, vanilla, egg and yoghurt in a bowl.

2 Stir in the remaining ingredients and mix until just blended.

3 Transfer the mixture into a 23 cm (9 in) square lightly oiled cake tin.

4 Bake at 180°C/350°F/gas mark 4 for 25–30 minutes until it is firm and springy to the touch.

Variations

• Chocolate Orange: omit the bananas and add the grated rind and juice of 2 oranges.

• Double Chocolate Chip: omit 1 banana and add 50 g (2 oz) chocolate chips or broken chocolate pieces.

Per serving (1 slice)		% energy
Energy	136 kcal	
Protein	3.4 g	10%
Fat	3.6 g	24%
Carbohydrate	24 g	66%
Fibre	1.4 g	

CHOCOLATE COCOA CAKE

My all-time favourite recipe for chocolate cake – it tastes like sheer heaven yet is unbelievably low in fat!

Makes 16 slices

350 g (12 oz) self raising flour (half wholemeal/half white)
6 tbsp cocoa, sieved
1 tsp salt
200 g (7 oz) brown sugar
1 tsp vanilla
4 tbsp oil
2 eggs
1 carton (125 g) plain yoghurt
300 ml (½ pint) skimmed milk

1 Combine the flour, cocoa, salt and sugar together in a bowl.
2 Add the remaining ingredients and mix well.
3 Transfer into a lightly oiled 18 × 28 cm (7 × 11 in) baking tin. Bake at 180°C/350°F/gas mark 4 for 25–30 minutes until golden. When cool, cut into slices.

Variations

• Chocolate Date Cake: add 75 g (3 oz) chopped dates to the mixture.
• Chocolate Chip Chocolate Cake: add 75 g (3 oz) chocolate chips to the mixture.
• Chocolate Raisin Cake: add 75 g (3 oz) raisins (or sultanas) to the mixture.

LOW FAT CHOCOLATE BROWNIES

Traditional brownies consist mainly of butter, chocolate and sugar – a high fat nightmare. This healthier version has the fat content substantially reduced and the chocolate replaced by cocoa and yoghurt.

Makes 16 squares

75 g (3 oz) self raising white flour
40 g (1½ oz) cocoa powder
175 g (6 oz) castor sugar
100 g (4 fl oz) vanilla yoghurt
2 eggs
1 tsp vanilla essence
1½ tbsp oil

1 Sift the flour and cocoa into a bowl. Add the remaining ingredients and mix together.
2 Spoon the mixture into a lightly oiled 20 cm (8 in) square baking tin and bake at 180°C/350°F/gas mark 4 for approximately 25 minutes, until springy to the touch.
4 Cool and cut into squares.

CAKES

Per serving (1 slice)		% energy
Energy	166 kcal	
Protein	4.1 g	10%
Fat	4 g	22%
Carbohydrate	30 g	68%
Fibre	1.8 g	

Per serving (1 brownie)		% energy
Energy	95 kcal	
Protein	2.2 g	9%
Fat	2.5 g	23%
Carbohydrate	17 g	68%
Fibre	0.5 g	

CAKES

CHOCOLATE FUDGE BROWNIES

This low fat version of brownies uses puréed prunes to replace the fat; surprisingly you can't taste the prunes at all and they keep the brownies wonderfully moist. Prune purée also contains fibre, iron, vitamin A and potassium.

Makes 16 squares

100 g (4 oz) plain chocolate
100 g (4 oz) prunes
3 tbsp water
3 egg whites
200 g (7 oz) light brown sugar
1 tsp salt
1 tsp vanilla essence
65 g (2½ oz) plain flour
25 g (1 oz) chopped walnuts
(optional)

1 Melt the chocolate in a bowl placed over a saucepan of simmering water.

2 Purée the prunes with the water in a liquidiser or food processor until roughly smooth.

3 In a bowl, mix together the prune purée, egg whites, sugar, salt and vanilla essence.

4 Add the melted chocolate and stir until smooth.

5 Fold in the sieved flour.

6 Spread the mixture into a lightly oiled 15 cm (6 in) square tin. Sprinkle with the walnuts, if applicable.

7 Bake at 180°C/350°F/gas mark 4 for 1 hour. When cool, cut into squares.

Per serving (1 brownie)		% energy
Energy	118 kcal	
Protein	1.5 g	5%
Fat	2.3 g	17%
Carbohydrate	24 g	78%
Fibre	0.8 g	

RESOURCES

Further Reading

The Complete Guide to Sports Nutrition (3rd ed)	Bean, A. (2000) A & C Black.
The Complete Guide to Strength Training (2nd ed)	Bean, A. (2001) A & C Black.
Power Eating (2nd edition)	Kleiner S. M. (2001) Human Kinetics.
Eat 5	Foster, H. (2002) Hamlyn.
Endurance Sports Nutrition	Girard Eberle, S. (2000) Human Kinetics.
Eat Smart Play Hard	Applegate, L. (2001) Rodale.
The Calorie, Carb & Fat Bible	Weight Loss Resources (2002).

Useful Addresses

British Nutrition Foundation	52–4 High Holborn, London WC1V 6RQ.
British Dietetic Association	5th Floor, Charles House, 148–9 Great Charles Street, Queensway, Birmingham B3 3HT, www.bda.uk.com.
Dietitians in Sport and Exercise Nutrition	PO Box 22360, London W13 9FL.
Eating Disorders Association	1st floor, Wensum House, 103

	Prince of Wales Road, Norwich, NR1 1DW, www.edauk.com.
Food Standards Agency	Room 621, Hannibal House, PO Box 30080, Elephant and Castle, London SE1 6YA, www.foodstandards.gov.uk.
Health Development Agency	Trevelyan House, 30 Great Peter Street, London SW1P 2HW, www.had-online.org.uk.
Health Supplements Information Service	Bury House, 126–8 Cromwell Road, London SW7 4ET, www.hsis.org.
The National Sports Medicine Institute of the United Kingdom	32 Devonshire Street, London W1G 6P, www.nsmi.org.uk.
Vegetarian Society	Parkdale, Dunham Road, Altrincham, Cheshire, WA14 4QG, www.vegsoc.org
Women's Nutritional	PO Box 268, Lewes, East Sussex BN7 1QN, *Advisory Service* www.wnas.org.uk.

On-Line Resources

www.nutrition.org.uk	The website of the British Nutrition Foundation provides nutrition fact sheets, information, educational resources and briefing papers.
www.USDA.gov	The website of the US Department of Agriculture contains useful and authoritative nutritional information.
www.phys.com	This website helps you work out your ideal weight, body fat percentage and calorie, fat, protein and carbohydrate needs.

237

www.mayohealth.org	The website of the famous Mayo clinic has an excellent food and nutrition section.
www.nutrio.com	A US website that provides up to date nutrition news, diet and fitness plans, menus and recipes.
www.webmd.com	This comprehensive US website has a directory of food topics and advice on many aspects of nutrition and fitness.

INDEX

Notes